T5-CVG-966

ONE STEP AHEAD

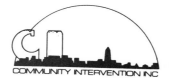

Community Intervention, Inc.
529 South Seventh Street
Suite 570
Minneapolis, Minnesota 55415
612/332-6537
800-328-0417

ONE STEP AHEAD

Early-Intervention Strategies
for
Adolescent Drug Problems

Joseph A. Muldoon ● James F. Crowley

Editors: *Pamela Eyden, Reggie McLeod, Kathleen Michels*
Photography: *Jeff Grosscup, Joe Muldoon, Barbara Nelson*
Typesetting: *Sexton Printing Co.*
Printing: *Sexton Printing Co.*

Library of Congress Catalog Number: 85-073646
ISBN: 0-9613416-1-0

Teenage drug and alcohol abuse means many things to many people. To educators it is, at the very least, an infraction of regulations and an intrusion into the educational process. To juvenile justice officials, it is a violation of the law and a precursor to other illegal activities. To parents it is a refutation of their basic values, a public embarrassment and a terrifying threat to the health and well-being of their children. To the politically ambitious, it can be a handy campaign issue—a matter of "law-and-order" with an apparently simple solution.

To kids, the use of alcohol and other drugs is a way to feel good, to have fun, to mask pain or to excuse behavior.

No single point of view encompasses the entire scope of the problem or provides a sound base for effective action. No individual can make a community aware of its problems, motivate others to attack those problems and coordinate the multitude of specific tasks needed to effect real changes. But, collectively, people can make a difference. Creative conflict among concerned people can help focus and refine our efforts. A diverse group of people who have a wide variety of skills can bring greater expertise to our projects. Broad participation also creates a strong base of support for bringing about change.

The solution to drug problems has much to do with how we relate to one another as human beings. Those who care, and care enough to become competent, find many rewards in their work and save many people years of suffering. Adults who join together to fight drug problems help not only the young people in their communities but themselves as well.

Table of Contents

Acknowledgments

Honest criticism shared with concern is a
jewel to the receiver. A rare jewel at that.
We have been fortunate to have had a
number of knowledgeable, involved, caring
people review our work, make criticisms
and offer suggestions. All of these people
have been invaluable to our efforts: Frank
Barr, consultant in public education and
former superintendent of the Fairview Park,
Ohio, Public Schools; Paul Dybvig, drug
education specialist for the Minnesota
Department of Education; Kirsten Dawson,
chemical education coordinator for the
Mounds View, Minnesota, Public Schools;
Barbara Jacobson, chemical health counselor for the Minneapolis Public Schools;
Gary Bowman, trainer, consultant and
therapist; and Tom Shroyer, professional
trainer and consultant in the field of early-
intervention programming for adolescents.
Helen Peterson, Mary Lou Jensen, Kathryn
McMonigal, Mary Lou Kosar and Gary
Swedberg also shared their knowledge
about special counseling techniques for
early intervention.

Mary Hoopman, resource specialist for
the Minneapolis Public Schools' Chemical
Awareness Program, contributed greatly to
Chapter Nine by collecting and assisting in
the analysis of data from the Minneapolis
program. Martin Remus, chemical dependency counselor for the Hennepin County,
Minnesota, Access Unit, and Mary Kelley,
director of the Hennepin County Access
Unit, provided invaluable data concerning
the assessment and referral processes of
their agency. Mike Andert, special education teacher for the Minnetonka, Minnesota, Public Schools, drew on his seven
years of personal experience in early-
intervention programming to offer suggestions on the Insight interview and Insight
Group format provided in the Appendix.

Pamela Eyden is the book's editor and
production manager. Without her honest
criticism the manuscript would never have
been completed; without her persistent
prodding the book would never have been
printed. Reggie McLeod's and Kathleen
Michels' copy editing helped make the book
as readable and error free as possible. Dolly
Gove's magic with computers helped trans-
form the tattered shreds of our edited
manuscript into a finely ordered document
ready for publication.

Introduction

Early intervention is a concept easily understood in general terms but, almost by definition, difficult to isolate and describe in a particular instance. Any action that is "early" is early only in relation to something else, an event or a condition that might have befallen a person had not some action been taken to change the course of events. When we help a young person who is becoming harmfully involved with alcohol or other mood-altering chemicals, it may never be entirely clear just what is being avoided, prevented or nipped in the bud.

Certainly there are those young people who, without some type of intervention, will become more and more involved with drugs and eventually become chemically dependent. Many others, rather than developing chronic drug dependencies, will feel the effects in terms of loss and regret: the competent athlete who throws away an opportunity to be a star; the shy person who does not use these years of intense social activity to learn how to meet and become friends with others; the lively, rebellious person whose last few years at home, rather than being a time of excitement and discovery, are filled with anger, pain and mutual recrimination. And there are, of course, those who will kill or be killed in drug-related automobile accidents.

Yes, some drug problems do resolve themselves, but how they are resolved and at what cost is of concern to us all.

Early intervention has implications not only for the ways young people learn to avoid harmful use of alcohol and other drugs but also for the ways in which schools and other community institutions and agencies resolve their "drug problems." Sometimes these problems remain unattended for so long that a lopsided overreaction gains well-meaning advocates in the community. Undercover police are sent in to gather information on unsuspecting students; arrests are made; young people, whose apprehension was a matter of chance (as was the nondetection of a great many others) are fined, sentenced, expelled from school and sent to juvenile detention centers for punishment. Clearly, it is important to intervene before the harmful consequences of *adult reactions* to drug problems ruin, if not people's entire lives, at least significant periods of their lives.

Early intervention, as we will describe it, is both simple and subtle. It is a process already being conducted successfully by groups of dedicated adults and young people who are, on the whole, neither softhearted dreamers nor unyielding cynics. These people are learning to be firm without being rigid, to be tough without being punitive. They are learning to help young drug abusers become aware of their problems, responsibilities and options without coddling or cursing them.

These people are tired of combating drug and alcohol abuse on a piecemeal, crisis-oriented basis. Tired of short-term programs designed as though the hard-won experience of others in the field—those who have succeeded *and* those who have failed—is totally irrelevant to the present situation. Tired of seeing their programs barely get off the ground before a new and different crisis comes along. Tired of always being one step behind the kids, the drugs, the pushers.

They are tired, but they have been learning. They have shown us that we *can* intervene before problems reach the crisis stage, and we *can* be well prepared for crises if and when they occur. We can stay *one step ahead*, ready, willing and able to help whenever we are needed.

A *coming of age*

Early intervention for drug problems has come of age. In the past we used the term "drug program" in a vague, undefined way. Check an article on a school "drug program" and you may find anything from an education-oriented prevention program to a program focused exclusively on aftercare for young people who have been through treatment for chemical dependency.

In preparing this book we looked at the bewildering proliferation of drug and alcohol programs, assessed their key components and forged them into an effective working model for reaching young people in ways appropriate for community-wide implementation.

Early-intervention programs for adults have already proved effective. Beginning as loosely organized "alcohol programs" that brought some simple self-help group concepts into the workplace, they have evolved into the more refined, efficient and effective "employee assistance" model. Using a well-developed employee assistance model as a reference point, program planners in the workplace no longer have to argue about whether or not a "drug program" can work. Rather, they can focus on specific factors that impede or facilitate the program's success, such as how well the program identifies employees in need; how effective it is in prompting them to come forward to ask for help or to accept help when it is offered; how successful it is in encouraging supervisors to follow appropriate procedures when confronting employees

whose work performance is lacking.

The employee assistance model has evolved from vague generalities to workable, nuts-and-bolts components. Similarly, early-intervention programs for young people can be planned, developed and evaluated in a conceptually sound, methodical fashion. This is not to say that early-intervention programs for young people are simply replications of the adult employee assistance model. Far from it. There are important distinctions to be made.

In *One Step Ahead* we consider the essential components of programs designed specifically for young people. We focus attention on how schools, courts, social service systems and specialized youth-oriented agencies can use this framework to define their needs and design programs. Our model also allows these diverse institutions and agencies to maximize their individual potentials for identifying, assessing and referring for help those young people who have drug-related and other disruptive personal problems.

Intended audiences

One Step Ahead is written primarily for people who have already made an investment in solving the drug and alcohol problems in their schools, agencies or communities. It is written for people who have read some of the current literature on alcohol and other drugs but who still seek a way to put these diverse insights and concepts into action. Educators, juvenile court personnel and social service professionals, whether working in direct service or administration, will find the book relevant to their needs. For program planners it offers a blueprint for the beginning stages of early-intervention planning and for checking program development. For those working directly with young people it offers an opportunity to see how the pieces fit together in the early-intervention process and how their jobs mesh with the jobs of others.

One Step Ahead can also be used, in whole or in part, by community task force members who want to assess what services are being offered, how well they are delivered and what services are missing from the community. Parents who are interested in developing services, not only for their own children but for all young people in their communities, will find the book helpful, as will agency board members who are hoping to nudge their program staff into looking at new ways of dealing with an old problem.

A *realistic approach*

When the subject of innovative early-intervention programming for drug problems is raised, professionals in social service or educational systems often protest, "We already have a person who deals with drug problems" or "Our state agency or the federal government already has consultants to take care of this."

Yes, it is true that various local and state agencies have mandates to "help all families and young people suffering from the problems of drug abuse" and yes, it is true that the federal government has mandated child-study teams or childcare teams to identify and help young people whose problems interfere with their education or social development. All these programs must be looked at closely as we attempt to develop a comprehensive, systems-oriented approach to early intervention. Some are of considerable assistance to those in need, others are useless.

Schools and social service agencies do not always operate in accord with the edicts of government bureaucracies and the ideals described in graduate school programs and textbooks. In discussing plans for early-intervention activities, we must take into account the mundane realities of everyday life. We know that some young people use drugs and still maintain their grade levels, thus eluding efforts to identify them solely on the basis of academic performance. We realize that some parents are prepared to fight the schools and the courts to the death, quite literally, to defend their children's "right" to use alcohol and other mood-altering chemicals. We are aware that youths have undergone unnecessary chemical dependency treatment and that some treatment centers, while operating ethically for the most part, do have a vested interest in running their programs at full capacity. We have also heard reports that teachers have been fired for becoming too interested in drug problems (which some administrators do not want to have discussed in public) and that local councils on alcoholism often do not get along with the youth counseling services or the drug abuse agencies in their areas. All these common, but frequently unstated, problems can adversely affect the operation of an early-intervention program if they go unrecognized.

Furthermore, even the best early-intervention programs have definite limitations. They cannot and should not try to do everything. A well-run program can eliminate much of the serious drug abuse and dependency in a community, but not all of it. Early-intervention programs cannot replace other efforts to deal with the problems. Parents must enforce limits, police must enforce laws, and schools must continue to enforce regulations. If the limits, laws and regulations are mutually compatible and if the consequences for violations are appropriate and humane, the additional efforts of an early-intervention program can be most effective.

One subject not covered in this book is the politics of programming—how to develop and maintain support for programs on an intra-agency and community-wide basis. The techniques and actions necessary to create the community support needed to establish early-intervention and related programs are encompassed in the process of *community mobilization* described by James Crowley in *Alliance for Change*.

We believe that early intervention is and
will continue to be one of the most effective
approaches ever developed for dealing with
both adolescent and adult drug and alcohol
problems. The viability of this new, ex-
panding field depends on each and every
one of us to review our experiences, to
refine our techniques and to share our
successes and failures with others. *One Step
Ahead* is the beginning, not the end, of the
sharing process. Future work in program
evaluation and research will greatly contribute to our ability to redirect people
toward happier, more fruitful lives.

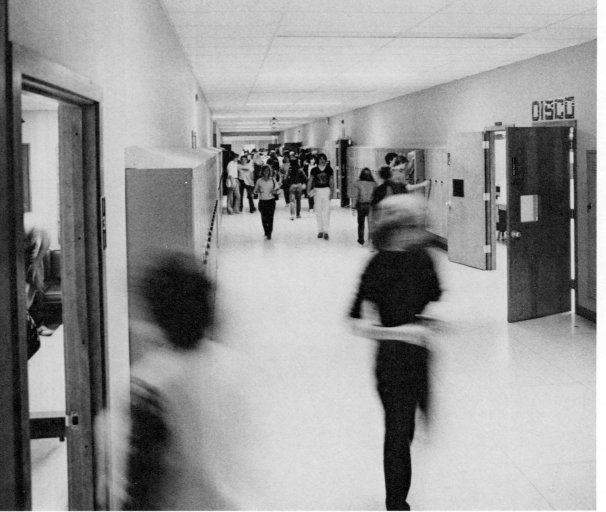

photo: Jeffrey Grosscup

CHAPTER ONE

FINDING OUR FOCUS
Basic Early-Intervention Processes

Imagine yourself floating in a hot-air balloon over Minneapolis, Minnesota, at mid-morning on a school day. Equipped with sophisticated optical and audio equipment, you are able to observe a wide variety of activities in the city's schools. In the far corner of the parking lot of one school, a student tells her boyfriend that she will not smoke marijuana with him before class anymore and even suggests that he ask their chemical awareness program counselor about getting some help for himself. In the group room of the counseling office, five students who have recently returned from treatment for drug problems hold their midweek support group meeting. In the office two doors down, a counselor talks to a student and her parents. After reviewing the girl's school records and a recent report that she had been intoxicated at a football game, the counselor urges the parents *not* to send their daughter immediately into chemical dependency treatment and explains why family counseling at a community agency is called for instead.

Later in the day a number of faculty members meet for inservice training on the problems of child abuse and family drug problems. An administrator standing near a computer reviews the quarterly data on the chemical awareness program. In the evening, groups of parents hold several meetings and school board members listen to a special presentation on the program.

At day's end, you might well wonder whether these wide-ranging activities are based on the "shotgun" approach to programming ("Let's try everything and see what works,") or on a comprehensive and coherent strategy.

In some school districts a few creative and highly energetic people have accomplished a great deal using the "shotgun" approach. By surviving a period of trial-and-error, hit-and-miss programming, some have managed to pull the results of their efforts together into a loosely defined master strategy. Unfortunately, the many handicaps inherent in this approach to programming usually cause the programs to falter and die out at about the same rate as the energetic people burn out. It is difficult to integrate other people into such programs, to make the fragmented, experimental ideas fit together efficiently and to obtain useful feedback on pilot-program results.

Careful planning can eliminate these handicaps. Indeed, the activities of successful early-intervention programs, like those of the

Minneapolis schools, are chosen or eliminated not by chance or whim but by careful consideration of the basic processes of early intervention.

The Processes of Early Intervention

Early-intervention programs can be set up in any youth-oriented agency or institution. Because, as will be discussed later, schools offer the most comprehensive systems for carrying out early-intervention programs, we use examples from schools. We do not mean to imply that schools are the only appropriate place for early-intervention programs or that schools are the best place for intervention with every type of young person. Court services, welfare and child protection units, mental health centers, churches, and specialized youth-oriented agencies all must contribute crucial early-intervention services—if not comprehensive early-intervention programs—to the continuum of care offered in the community.

An early-intervention program for adolescent drug problems encompasses the following six key processes:

▪ *Identification*. Staff members, young people, parents and others must be able to recognize patterns of behavior commonly related to drug use or other personal problems. They must also understand that the services of the early-intervention program can help alleviate such problems.

▪ *Initial action*. When a youth has a problem with alcohol or other drugs, there are a variety of ways to initiate early intervention. She or he may ask for help, but more often it is an adult who takes the first step. For example, a teacher may talk to the student to clarify a situation concerning academic performance or attendance; consult with a person working in the early-intervention program; refer the student directly to a school administrator for disciplinary action; or make a referral to a counselor for help. The step taken depends on the specific policies and procedures of the school.

The many barriers to initial action must be carefully considered. It is extremely important to differentiate problems of identification from problems of initial action. Those who have identified a youth with drug problems or other disruptive personal problems will be much more likely to take initial action if the steps are simple and concrete. If, for example, teachers know that they only have to dial a well-publicized number for consultation when *any* problem arises, they are more likely to take that step. If, on the other hand, teachers are expected to check out state laws on drug use, to decide whether or not the current situation requires action, and then to determine exactly which action must be taken, the initial move toward intervention might well be stifled by indecision and inertia.

▪ *Preliminary assessment*. When a problem concerning a young person's drug use arises, someone must obtain information about his or her general behavior and specific drug-related activities and make sure that he or she understands the situation and the options. A counselor or pre-assessment team must also determine whether or not referral to an outside agency is necessary. The assessment is called "preliminary" because no diagnosis of physical or emotional illness is made. It is presumed that before any agency places a young person in therapy or treatment for drug abuse or other disruptive personal problems, an in-depth assessment will be conducted to determine the most appropriate course of action. A major part of the preliminary assessment is *data gathering*. If the front-line people—adults who have daily contact with young people in educational, work or recreational activities—contribute willingly to the data-gathering process, the task of preliminary assessment is much easier.

▪ *Referral to appropriate services*. Sometimes a youth can benefit from group counseling or other activities provided by the institution or agency where the problem was first identified. Sometimes, however, the situation calls for more in-depth assessment or treatment. Making the right referral to an appropriate service at the right time is crucial to the early-intervention process. Who is referred where and at what point in the process depends on organizational priorities; availability of funds; motivation of the young person and parents; and many other factors. Referral patterns can reveal much about the nature of an early-intervention program.

▪ *Appropriate use of a continuum of care.* The continuum of care includes all services available to assist young people and their families in dealing with the problems uncovered in the early-intervention process. A few preliminary assessment and short-term counseling services can be offered by the early-intervention agent, but most necessary counseling and treatment services fall outside the domain of the schools and courts. Ongoing communication and cooperation among a wide range of service providers greatly improve the effectiveness of early-intervention programs. Mutual agreements regarding criteria for referral and clear-cut procedures for the sharing of confidential information are crucial to providing appropriate, coordinated services to young people.

In this book we do not address the development of adequate counseling and treatment services in detail because this, obviously, is a vast subject. The types of services available, however, are such a key factor in how an early-intervention program functions that they must be considered part of the early-intervention process.

▪ *Support in maintaining changes.* Whether young people are treated for drug problems on an inpatient or outpatient basis, regular support is needed to help them with the changes they are attempting to make. The place where a young person is identified as having a drug problem, such as a school or community recreation center, is often the place where the pressure to use drugs is most intense. Although many agencies must be involved in the support network, support offered within high-pressure settings can greatly aid in helping young people stay drug free. Many treatment professionals name support groups in the schools as the single most important factor in keeping kids off drugs after they leave treatment.

A brief review of the basic processes is helpful in assessing existing programs. For instance, if a school program has no active identification process and referrals are primarily an offshoot of the disciplinary process, the effect on the number and types of students involved in the program will be evident. For the most part, these programs are playing a catch-up game and cannot be expected to intervene with a representative cross section of students who have problems with alcohol or other drugs. The types of students reached are determined by activities outside of the early-intervention program rather than by the program itself.

Keeping program processes constantly in mind helps avoid many fruitless arguments during planning and provides for more flexibility and creativity in problem solving. If, for example, a program is not being used by students, a global statement like "Drug programs just don't work in our community" does nothing to resolve the situation. An investigation to determine which specific objectives are not being met can, on the other hand, make a world of difference. It may be that staff members and students have no trouble identifying problems but do not take any action because they have heard that program services are not helpful. In this case, attempts to resolve the problem of low utilization of services by pumping out more information on drugs or family problems will do nothing. In fact, they may only reinforce the opinion that "School programs don't work."

Dealing with Conflict

Problems surrounding adolescent drug use invariably draw out many conflicting attitudes, opinions and facts from those seeking to make things better for young people.

Conflict need not have negative results, however. It can make us more aware of problems, encourage change and increase our motivation to deal with longstanding deficiencies in our organizations. In order to resolve conflicts to the benefit of all concerned, conflict must be managed well. Some suggestions for dealing with conflict are:

○ Recognize that conflict is normal and inevitable. Whenever two or more gather together to perform a task, there will be some conflict over goals or methods. Conflict does *not* mean that there is something wrong with the people or the organizations they are working in.

○ Make your organization a safe place for dealing with conflict. Allow people to have differences of opinion and to express these differences clearly. Some organizations make it clear that conflict and controversy are valued and not seen as a threat to the organization.

○ Define the conflict clearly. Separate personal issues from organizational issues; separate problems over goals from problems over methods.

○ Emphasize areas of agreement as well as areas of disagreement. Emphasize areas where trust exists even when a lack of trust must be noted.

○ Avoid polarization. Do not allow conflicts to come down to a "win-lose," "either-or" choice. There are often many alternative resolutions for any one conflict and a variety of alternatives should be explored before decisions are made.

○ Use a clearly recognized, accepted structure for decision-making. If an organization is autocratic, with a chief executive making decisions with input from other people, that type of conflict resolution is acceptable. If an organization is supposed to be democratic, then a democratic structure should be used to resolve conflicts.

A clear focus on the six processes of early intervention can also help resolve philosophical arguments about who should conduct programs. For example, some people may argue that early intervention into drug problems is a job for mental health centers, not schools. This argument could last for years, but it can be short-circuited by a practical, nuts-and-bolts consideration of how children who use drugs can most effectively be identified, assessed and referred for help. Communities *can* center their early-intervention programs in mental health agencies. However, they must realize that by doing so they may be limiting both the number and, depending on the agency's mission and image in the community, the types of young people likely to be identified.

We refer to the six early-intervention processes throughout this book. Their full significance will gradually become more clear as various program details and issues are discussed in relation to them. *One Step Ahead* concludes with a review of these basic processes and guidelines for using them in program evaluation.

Challenging Our Assumptions About Drug Use

Analysis of the six processes shows why early-intervention programs cannot focus exclusively on chemically dependent young people. Chemical dependency per se cannot be identified by teachers or other adults working with young people. These front-line adults can identify behaviors that may be related to drug use and a range of personal problems, but in most cases a preliminary assessment and a full-scale professional assessment must precede the *diagnosis* of chemical dependency. For every chemically dependent young person who is identified, many other nondependent drug users and victims of child abuse will also come to light.

Once identified, disruptive personal problems must be addressed. This does not mean that early-intervention programs must provide extensive in-house services for all disruptive personal problems. Generally, schools find it efficient to offer some intervention and support services for young drug users, but they seldom offer groups specifically for youths who are being battered or sexually abused. Such problems are immediately referred for intervention by other services in the community, although school counselors usually stay in contact with these young people to offer support. Also, because treatment for child abuse may involve some disruption of a student's routine, a caring adult should be available in the school to help with scheduling conflicts and problems caused by missed schoolwork.

Because they inevitably encountered a wide range of drug and family problems, most alcoholism programs in business and industry had to switch from a narrowly focused alcohol problems model to a broad-based employee assistance model. The argument was not whether alcoholism is or is not the most serious impediment to job performance—in many occupations it probably is—but whether it was ethical or practical to ignore other problems once they were uncovered. The situation is the same in youth-oriented drug-intervention programs.

Many adults working with young drug abusers see only a specific population of young people. These adults may have done volunteer work in a halfway house for chemically dependent teenagers, served as juvenile probation officers or worked in psychiatric settings. Each of these contexts provides a different view of the drug problem. Those who have worked in an inpatient hospital treatment program may view early intervention as a method of seeking out chemical dependency. Those from a court setting may judge a problem by how much illegal behavior is associated with it. Those from the field of psychiatry may assume that drug abuse does not exist without psychiatric dysfunction. People who have not had contact with the families of young drug abusers have little comprehension of the many obvious and subtle ways in which family members affect one another's use of alcohol and other drugs.

When people turn their focus from a specific population in a given treatment or correctional program to the large population of young people addressed by early-intervention programs, it is very easy for them to presume that all the young people they encounter are similar to those in treatment settings. This is a false assumption that can have serious implications, especially if, on its strength alone, young people are immediately labeled chemically dependent, emotionally disturbed or incorrigible before other possibilities have been considered.

This is not a philosophical argument. It does not boil down to whether or not we *believe* severe drug abuse is a disease or merely a symptom of other, more serious problems. It does not depend on whether or not we want to work with only the most severely impaired young people. It cannot be swept aside by saying, "Well, there are many kinds of drug problems, but we will deal only with a particular type of drug problem." The very nature of the early-intervention process and the breadth and depth of drug use behaviors necessitate our working with all kinds of drug problems as well as other personal problems.

It is easy to make assumptions about kids who use drugs. Some people want to write them off as "losers" and some want to believe they are completely different from the "jocks" or the "intellectuals." When a naive and frightened drug user attempts to be seen as "cool" and "together," equally naive professionals depict them as "streetwise" or as "psychopaths." In fact, kids who have problems with drugs come in a variety of shapes, sizes and personalities, and most carry a good-sized package of pain with them.

For some teenagers, drugs are *the* major problem in their lives, the source of most of their troubles. For others, it is not so simple. They may have had serious problems before they started using drugs, problems that subsequently became worse.

Clearly, kids try drugs for different reasons, have different reactions to drugs and must be treated in different ways. There is one constant, however. The more they use, the more their problems—severe emotional problems, normal problems of growing up or simple boredom—become deeply enmeshed with and tightly bonded to their drug use, which may, if it has not already happened, take on a life of its own.

The Need for a System-wide Approach

The six processes of early intervention may seem overly analytical to some people, and some competent counselors may well wonder why they should even consider them. Why not just continue working on a personal, case-by-case basis? If you feel this way, as did both authors at one time, consider the fact that drug abuse does not exist in a vacuum. The origins of drug problems and the conditions that actively or passively perpetuate these problems lie not only with individuals but also within systems: families, schools, communities and the entire culture.

To be effective, early intervention must be conducted on a system-wide basis. One teacher will have greater success in confronting a problem of poor attendance if all teachers do the same. A counselor trying to make a preliminary assessment of a young person's problems will find the task easier if there are established procedures for gathering information and guidelines for making decisions. Parents whose children are referred to some service in the community will be less likely to feel mistreated if they know that other

Demonstrations of Program Effectiveness

The following areas are often cited to demonstrate the benefits of an early-intervention program: identification of students with drug problems; satisfaction with program services; reduction of drop-out rate; financial advantages; and the powerful effect of primary treatment programs on chemically dependent students.

○ *Identification of problem students*. Clearly, early-intervention programs in schools have been successful in identifying students with drug problems. Statistics from an unpublished annual report of the Minneapolis Public Schools indicate that in one school year (1983-84) personnel from the chemical awareness program offered assistance to 1,426 of the district's 17,442 secondary students. In a nearby suburban district with a secondary enrollment of 8,000 students, 6% received preliminary screening or assessment services in one year. Therefore, since most students who complete junior and senior high school are involved in secondary education for six years, it is possible that in a given school district as many as one quarter to one third of all secondary students will undergo some type of basic screening assessment. (An in-depth statistical analysis of the Minneapolis program is presented in Chapter Nine.)

Data also show that, in order to identify troubled youths, schools and other agencies do not have to rely strictly on the apprehension of young people who violate laws on drug possession or use. Self-referrals, referrals by friends and referrals by family members account for a large percentage of the young people who receive services.

○ *Satisfaction with program services*. In one school's report on its early-intervention program (Larsen, 1982), 83.4% of 62 students who received services rated the program "excellent" or "very good"; none rated it less than "fair."

More important, perhaps, are the high ratings given by teachers concerning student behavior: 78% said that "in-class behavior is improved"; 75% indicated that attendance improved; 36% noted that tardiness had been reduced; and 61% reported that students who had participated in the program showed "improved scholastic performance." In regard to the overall performance of the program in the high school, 67% of the staff members rated the program "excellent" or "very good," while only 3% rated it less than "fair."

○ *Reduction of drop-out rate*. Many program coordinators

believe that intervention/prevention programs can significantly reduce the drop-out rate among students who abuse drugs. They also acknowledge that they have a long way to go to prove their case because no hard data currently exist in this area. There are, however, some favorable indications. The schools in Bloomington, Minnesota, reviewed the academic records of ten randomly selected seniors who were members of abstinence support groups (originally reported in *Community Intervention*, Fall 1982). Some of these seniors had been in treatment for chemical dependency, some had not. The records of this group were compared with those of nine randomly selected seniors who had been referred to the chemical awareness program but had not followed through on the action recommended. All the seniors who participated in the program graduated, whereas 55% of those who did not participate eventually dropped out of school. Although this finding certainly does not amount to scientific proof that the drug program was the key intervening varia-

continued on next page

ble, it has been accepted as a favorable indication of the usefulness of the student support group system.

○ *Financial advantages*. Most people familiar with the effects of severe drug abuse agree that a large number of students who have been identified as being harmfully involved with drugs would not attend school without some help. This is important given the fact that many states award grants to schools on the basis of average daily attendance.

In Minnesota, schools receive approximately $1,230 per student per year. If 50 students remain in school because of program efforts, the school can gain $61,500 per year in funding. If 75 students remain, $92,250 can be saved in state aid to the school. In many secondary schools with an enrollment of 6,000 or more, 75 to 100 students are involved in abstinence support groups.

Again, these data are speculative, based on early indications, not on hard, bottom-line, cost-benefit analysis. Nevertheless, even though aftercare or abstinence support groups are only one part of an overall intervention/prevention program, it is conceivable that in states where aid to schools is

dependent on school attendance, efforts to deal with the more serious problems of drug and alcohol abuse could pay for themselves.

○ *Effectiveness of primary treatment*. Although only a small percentage of students (1% to 2% in the programs we have reviewed) are actually referred for primary treatment from early-intervention programs each year, this group can have a powerful impact. School staff members are frequently very impressed when formerly disruptive students do a complete turnaround and become positive influences within the school.

One of the few truly intensive, government-sponsored evaluations of adolescent inpatient programs (Mitchell, 1977) concluded that such programs have a "profound effect on many of the patients" treated. Follow-up evaluations from the primary treatment unit of New Connection Programs, Inc., in St. Paul, Minnesota, indicated that six months after leaving treatment,

more than 95% of the program graduates studied had reduced or eliminated the use of drugs (65% were abstinent) and 95% were in school or working or both.

*   *   *

Except for the findings drawn from the articles by Mitchell and Larsen, which are listed in the bibliography, all other data used here were derived from the unpublished program reports of several early-intervention and treatment programs in the Minneapolis area. Our thanks to the following program administrators and researchers who shared information with us: Caroline Cade, Bloomington School District; Sylvia Horwitz Byrum, Robbinsdale School District; Dan Loewenson and Mary Hoopman, Minneapolis Public Schools; and Nancy Briggs, New Connection Programs, Inc.

parents' children have been treated in a similar manner. A probation officer will be more effective if all juvenile court judges make appropriate use of treatment services.

Failure to recognize the need for system-wide intervention has worn out many competent adults who work with young drug users. Adults who must work alone can do an excellent job with a few young people for a limited time. However, lack of understanding from their colleagues and service professionals, lack of consistency among educators and lack of cooperation from parents can make their efforts seem short-lived and hopeless. By establishing procedures for identification, initial action, preliminary assessment and referral, we bring coherence and consistency to our efforts.

Many adults working with young drug users have been able to accomplish a great deal because they have experience in direct service, they are competent and they care. Most of what has been done to help young drug users and their families is due to the efforts of loving, concerned "true believers"—people who believe in kids and in their own and their colleagues' fight against drug abuse. This question may then arise: If we stop talking about "helping those kids who are hurting" and begin trying to "develop effective early-intervention programs for young people," will we lose some of the enthusiasm and dedication needed to really help people in trouble?

In a word, no.

An empathetic understanding of the pain of young people and their families is extremely important. In fact, we go so far as to suggest that those reading this book in a detached, academic manner without a clear dedication to helping young people are unlikely to become consistent advocates of effective programming and agents of real change. Accurate empathy is important not only to the clinical worker but to those involved in general programming as well. That

is why, in *Alliance for Change*, James Crowley placed so much emphasis on the need for the kind of training that helps people develop empathy, concern and enthusiasm.

The Success of Early-Intervention Programs

The complexity of the drug problem may seem overwhelming, but it is not. We can recognize the multidimensional nature of adolescent drug use and take it into account without becoming scattered and unfocused. The model we present here is designed to deal with drug problems that differ from one another in degree and quality. Our model takes advantage of the strengths afforded by a mix of personalities and occupational roles. Teachers who teach well, who hold students accountable and who do not try to solve students' problems all by themselves are more helpful than those who attempt to alleviate drug problems on their own by using one-to-one counseling methods. Schools that refer students for outside help are more effective than those that repeatedly place students with serious drug problems in special education courses or offer an overabundance of chemical dependency services. Agencies that recognize they are better equipped to deal with adults and do not attempt to be all things to all people are more helpful than agencies that believe their model for dealing with alcoholism fits all kinds of problems related to alcohol and other drugs.

Proper conceptualization of issues related to drugs and the use of methodical approaches to programming have yielded definite gains in the struggle against drug problems. The effectiveness of early-intervention programs for adults is beyond question. Employee assistance and alcoholism programs in business and industry have clearly improved employee performance through intervention and treatment for alcoholism (Muldoon and Berdie, 1980).

Early-intervention programs for adolescents have not yet received the funding needed to perform in-depth evaluations similar to those done on employee assistance programs. Preliminary data indicate, however, that these programs are very effective in identifying students with problems; promoting staff and student satisfaction with program services; lowering drop-out rates; providing financial advantages to the school; and utilizing effective primary treatment services. (See "Demonstrations of Program Effectiveness" on page 13 for a detailed account of some of these preliminary findings.)

* * *   * * *   * * *

In this chapter we described, very briefly, the six processes of early intervention. Before we can really understand the implications of these processes in terms of the tasks before us, we have to consider in more detail just what this "drug problem" is. In the next chapter we discuss some key aspects of adolescent drug use and their implications for early intervention.

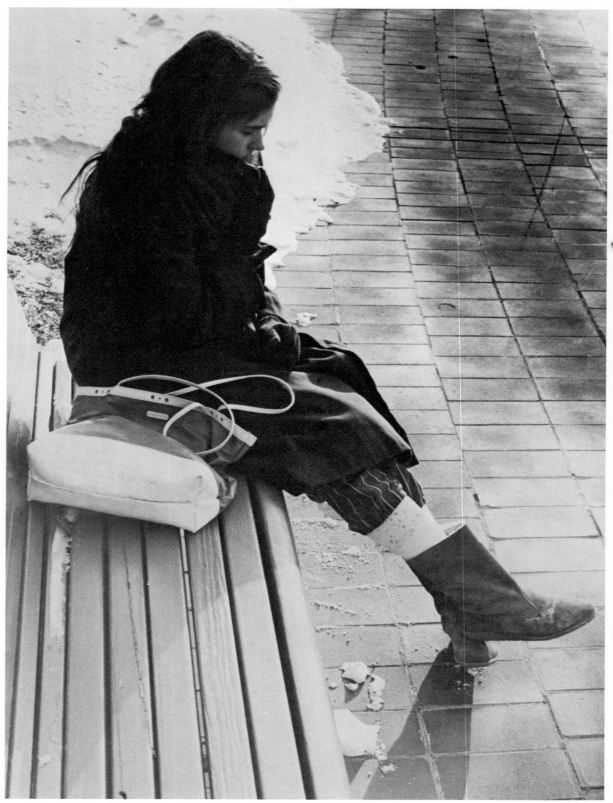

photo: Barbara Nelson

CHAPTER TWO

ADOLESCENT DRUG USE
From Controversy to Consensus

Conflict among practitioners and theore-ticians is a common problem in any new field. Fierce conflict in the field of adolescent chemical health/chemical dependency, though, has inhibited open discussion of the issues and made lonely people of many of us. There are, for instance, college professors who have been ridiculed by their intellectual colleagues for defending the effectiveness, for some people, of Alcoholics Anonymous. Treatment center counselors, out of fear of jeopardizing their careers, have occasionally stifled doubts about labeling some of their young drug-using clients alcoholic or chemi-cally dependent. Task forces have been fa-tally divided by unresolved conflicts over whether alcohol use is or is not as serious as the use of other drugs.

There are signs, however, that times are changing. Again and again, as we talked with professionals across the country, we found a new willingness to discuss the issues behind the conflicts. This comment from a counselor who performs preliminary assess-ments in a school program is typical: "During the first two years I was working in schools, it didn't occur to me to question whether or not a kid who used drugs was chemically depen-dent. I thought, 'Of course, he's dependent!' Now I see the need to consider—seriously consider—other possibilities."

Similarly, psychologists and psychiatrists seem willing to admit that traditional meth-ods of psychotherapy are not always effec-tive. They are recognizing the fact that when chemical use is an issue for an adolescent or a factor in a young person's family problems, it must be addressed directly and abstinence in-sisted upon.

Some of these conflicts are based on clear disagreement over matters of substance; oth-ers result from a poor definition of certain terms and concepts. Common points of con-fusion are:

o the question of the legality of the drug and the drug use;
o difficulty with the terms "use," "abuse" and "experimentation";
o disputes over "problems related to use" be-ing the sole criterion for intervention;
o definition of a "primary" illness or syn-drome;
o the "chemical dependency" concept; and
o the role of delusion and denial in drug problems.

In this chapter we look at each of these issues.

Illegal Drug Use and Use of Illegal Drugs

Whether drug use is "illegal drug use" de-pends which drug is used, who uses it and how it is used. Use of alcohol by a 15-year-old is illegal drug use. Until very recently anyone who used marijuana was guilty of illegal drug use; now some states allow this drug to be prescribed in special medical cases. Over-prescription of medications can contribute to drug abuse; however, it is not always illegal, just poor medical practice. Inhalants, such as glue and paint, can be bought by minors; using them to become intoxicated is illegal.

We do not often employ the term "use of illegal drugs" because it implies that we are not including misuse of various drugs, such as alcohol, that can be used legally under some circumstances. Even the term "illegal drug use," which takes into account the use of alcohol by minors, describes only a part of the drug and alcohol problem in our country. Among adults, most drug problems stem from legal use of the drug alcohol and many other problems result from excessive use of legally prescribed drugs.

Controversy Over Use, Abuse and Experimentation

The terms "use," "abuse" and "experimentation" are more useful and relevant in some contexts than in others. In regard to public policies and school regulations, it may not be helpful to distinguish between "drug use" and "drug abuse." In a great many situations it does not matter whether the person in possession or under the influence of a drug regularly uses, finds it difficult not to use or often behaves dangerously while using. If a person is not supposed to carry an open bottle of alcohol in the car or to have marijuana at all, then portions of public policies and school regulations that address those behaviors need make no distinction between a "drug user" and a "drug abuser." Whether the person in question has a problem with the drug does not matter and should not be taken into account when the legality or illegality of his or her actions is determined.

The situation changes drastically, however, when a specific youth in a specific situation is being assessed with regard to the possibility

of assistance for emotional, family or drug problems. If the assessors do not make a distinction between a person who merely uses drugs occasionally and a person who is physically and psychologically dependent on drugs, there is no possibility of developing effective intervention and treatment programs for drug problems.

No truly useful purpose is served by trying to establish specific criteria for applying such labels as "experimenter," "drug user" and "drug abuser." Even if one believes the concepts are valid, the specific cut-off points for deciding when a young person moves from experimenter to user to abuser would inevitably be arbitrary. Nevertheless, we do need to make some distinctions among the wide range of drug-use problems that require a range of interventions. Our need is pragmatic. For example, a young person may use alcohol or other drugs for several months with friends who are heavy drug users. When she or he is caught and sent to an assistant principal, a suspension may or may not result, but feelings of embarrassment, fear of not getting a scholarship and shame for having deceived parents may convince the student that using chemicals is not worth the risk. If abstinence continues it would be fair to assume that this student's drug problem is probably different from the drug problems of those who do not, will not or cannot stop after receiving a disciplinary reprimand.

One good way to start making valid and useful distinctions is by asking the following questions: "Does the person stop using drugs voluntarily or after a low-level intervention?" "Is the problem so deeply entrenched as to require more than disciplinary or legal sanctions?"

It may be said that young people who experiment with drugs and then quit after a low-level intervention have emerged unharmed. But the younger the person, the less likely the concept of "harmless experimentation" applies. It is not harmless experimentation, it is just dumb luck, if a group of 13-year-olds get drunk on their parents' liquor and do not hurt themselves or someone else or damage property.

Problems Related to Use

In referring to adults who abuse alcohol, we commonly use the terms "problem drinkers" and "alcoholics." Problem drinkers are those people who use alcohol in such amounts or with such frequency or behave in such ways while under the influence that it adversely affects their relationships, their physical condition or their abilities to carry out responsibilities. Some of these drinkers are alcoholics, i.e., they have a primary, progressive and chronic disease known as alcoholism. Some of them do not have this disease.

Labeling "problem drug users" is merely a matter of assigning a specific but arbitrary name to a certain portion of the range of people who have problems related to drug use. For some people, their main problem with drug use is trouble with the law. They may be angry young people who are rebelling in a variety of ways, only one of which is illegal drug use. Nonetheless, their drug use is creating ongoing problems. For others, drug use has caused them to seek out an entirely new group of drug-using friends, has led to a decline in school grades and, despite repeated attempts, has proved very difficult to stop. Both types of drug user may be considered "problem users," but they need significantly different services.

Not the sole criterion for intervention

We often hear it blithely stated that "problems related to use are the only basis schools have for intervention with a student. Illegal use of drugs, including underage alcohol use and misuse of prescription drugs, is not the school's or the therapist's concern." Taken at face value, such a statement has some common-sense appeal. There are, however, clear limits to the application of the "problems-related-to-use" criterion as the sole basis for intervention. For example, most people would not approve of an 11-year-old drinking a couple of beers two or three times a week, even if the precocious little devil were still going to school, doing as well as ever and not causing any problems at home. But what about a 14-year-old or a 16-year-old? At what age do we draw the line? At what age do we begin to focus on the existence of problems as the criterion for intervention? Given the tremendous variation in physical and emotional maturity among young people, the question is complex—so complex as to be unanswerable in most situations. For families, schools and communities, the only safe, reasonable and enforceable policy is no drug use by children or adolescents.

The argument that problems related to use are the only criterion for intervention proves problematical in other ways. Consider the 16-year-old who has an IQ of 120 and considerable talent for mathematics, who uses marijuana and alcohol together four times a week. If this student is able to progress academically at an average rate even while under the influence of drugs, should we allow him or her to come to class stoned? Hardly. Parents and educators have an investment in encouraging students to achieve their full potential, not simply rise to minimum standards. If students can perform well when high—some probably can, most probably cannot—they need greater challenges. Moreover, academic performance is not the only educational issue. We want students to find satisfaction in the learning experience itself and not have it distorted by drug use.

Drug use alone, then, can be a legitimate criterion for intervention. Problems related to drug use may be one criterion—along with frequency of use, quantity of drugs used and other factors—by which to determine the type of intervention called for, but it cannot be assumed that "non-problem drug use" is acceptable.

The "trickle-down effect"

Whenever people consider allowing older adolescents to use drugs as long as they use them "responsibly," they should consider the effect on younger siblings and friends. Many parents and professionals feel that a "trickle-down effect" surrounds legal alcohol use or generally accepted marijuana use. Whenever certain young people are allowed to use drugs, youths one or two years younger inevitably gain more access to those drugs. If 21-year-olds can drink, 19-year-olds have an easier time obtaining alcohol; if 15-year-olds are given tacit permission to use drugs "responsibly" or discreetly, 13-year-olds have a better chance of obtaining drugs.

Predicting future problems

The degree of problems with present use is not always predictive of future problems. Although young people who use drugs without *apparent* problems are more likely to slip through intervention systems than others, this does not mean that they will continue to avoid problems in the future. The way young people get into or avoid trouble when using drugs is often merely a manifestation of their personal styles. Those who tend to act out also tend to be rowdy or destructive when using drugs. Successful "family heroes" may continue to use drugs, especially alcohol, very heavily but quietly and become addicted before they realize that alcohol should be of any concern to them at all. The quiet, shy, ingratiating young lad whom everybody likes may be far ahead of his more disruptive peers in having a serious, long-term problem with drugs.

Family background also influences the way young people get into or avoid trouble when using drugs. Children of alcoholics are a case in point. Regardless of how obvious their problems with chemicals are when they first start using, such children run a greater risk of becoming chemically dependent than others (Vaillant and Milofsky, 1982).

Reasons for abstaining from drug use

The reasons for abstinence need not always be contingent on an absolute medical necessity. For some chemical dependency professionals, the issue of abstinence is inextricably entwined with their concept of the disease of alcoholism or drug addiction. "This kid has a chronic, progressive, incurable disease and is incapable of using alcohol or drugs without eventually losing control and suffering severe consequences," sayeth one. "This kid is not an alcoholic," quoth another, "so she has nothing to worry about."

In a given situation, either statement may be correct. Sometimes, however, the concepts become distorted. To motivate young clients to stay away from chemicals, a counselor may feel it is necessary to convince them that they have a chronic, incurable disease. Those professionals who reject a specific diagnosis or even the entire disease concept of alcoholism, may also reject the beneficial effects that abstinence can have on an adolescent's life. The following are just a few reasons why a particular young person, who may or may not be chemically dependent, would do well to refrain from chemical use:

■ *Immaturity*. A person may simply be too immature to use chemicals appropriately. Never mind that he or she is 21 years old and has some friends who drink appropriately. Other friends may be quite different. In time, he or she may change, but for now abstinence makes sense.

■ *Age*. Drug use at an early age can disrupt social and psychological development. It is also associated with long-term drug problems. As was noted previously, adults have the right to set clear standards based on age alone. No adolescent has to use mood-altering chemicals for recreational purposes.

■ *Assessment*. If a person has problems with drugs, abstinence facilitates assessment of the trouble spots in her or his life. How does she or he feel when not high? From where do those feelings come? Where will this lead in terms of treatment planning? Without abstinence, evaluation is more difficult. Furthermore, can he or she demonstrate the ability to stay away from drugs? If not, why not?

■ *Practical considerations*. A young person who has been in juvenile court twice for possession of marijuana has some kind of problem, either with the law or with the illegal drug. He or she needs to hear, "OK, so the cops have you fingered. Stay away from the drugs. They are not worth going to jail for. And if they *are*, then you've got a drug problem."

■ *Priority*. Abstinence may be a priority even if a person's drug use stems from some underlying psychological or emotional problem. Psychotherapy cannot proceed until drug use ceases. (This subject is discussed at greater length later.)

■ A *positive approach*. Attempting to control drug use may take more "air time" in a person's thoughts than it should. Deciding what is appropriate and what is not appropriate may just be more trouble than it is worth. Quite likely, in several years, such decisions will be easier to make. Abstinence allows young people in this situation to devote all their energy to natural highs and to work on the many important challenges facing them as they grow older.

"Symptomatic," "Primary" or "A Priority"?

Adolescent drug use, which is sometimes a primary problem and often the priority for immediate treatment, is not always both at the same time. There has long been controversy as to whether alcoholism in adults is a "primary disease." What is or is not a "disease" is a broad sociocultural issue as well as a medical issue. We will not pursue that issue here, but we will consider whether adolescent drug problems can be viewed as a primary problem, thus meriting intervention and treatment in its own right.

It is disheartening to see the amount of confusion, chaos and—dare we say it?—sloppy thinking on the issue of whether adolescent drug use must be labeled a primary illness or a symptom of other, more important problems. We hope to convince you that this dichotomy is by no means the only option and that these concepts are not necessarily the key determinants for deciding what action must be taken at a particular time.

Two or more primary problems are possible

A person can have more than one primary illness or primary problem. The term "primary" is an unfortunate one because it implies that to be so named a condition must be first in order or in time—"that from which others are derived" or "first in importance, chief in principle." These dictionary definitions have little bearing on the way in which people in the field use the term "primary." Most seem to mean that the disease, condition or syndrome in question is not currently dependent on another disease, condition or syndrome and would not disappear if the other did. Given such a definition, it is clear that a person can have two or more primary problems at the same time, such as a drug problem, a family problem and a behavioral problem. Two or three primary problems, while individually self-sustaining, can be mutually exacerbating. Family problems can make a drug problem worse, even if the drug problem is itself a primary, self-sustaining condition.

Symptoms can become primary problems

There are those who argue that adolescent drug use is merely a symptom of a primary problem, such as dysfunctional family relationships or inadequate self-concept and that wise treatment should focus on the primary problem. Symptoms, however, can become primary problems in themselves. If a person who smokes heavily seeks medical care because of shortness of breath, the physician could focus on this complaint and recommend weekly oxygen treatment and exercises to increase lung capacity. However, the physician is more likely to focus on the primary problem—addiction to nicotine—and advise the patient to quit smoking. In this example, treatment of the symptom rather than the primary problem would be foolish. However, if the patient was later found to have lung cancer, this disease would be a primary problem in itself. Treatment would then focus also on the cancer, not just on the cigarette smoking that caused it.

Similarly, adolescent drug use can quickly become a *functionally autonomous* problem, often one that is more serious than its precipitating causes. Those who have experience with adolescent drug abusers will probably have little difficulty accepting this. We ask those without such experience or those who remain skeptical to consider the possibility. Of course, even after the problem of drug use has been dealt with, the precipitating factors remain and merit intervention.

"Primary" and "priority" are two different concepts

It could be said of an epileptic who has broken many bones during violent seizures that the broken bones are secondary to the primary problem of severe epilepsy. However, when a bone breaks, the patient is not kept from emergency treatment because he or she is scheduled to attend a session of group counseling for epileptics or consult a pharmacologist about a change in medication. The priority in this case is to set the bone.

Similarly, even when very serious problems accompany drug use or are even the cause of drug use, the first priority for treatment may be to stop the drug use, since continued use will undermine other forms of therapy. For example, an abused child may need intensive treatment for psychological and behavioral problems, only one of which is drug use. If this drug use is not treated first, however, it

may interfere with any psychotherapy undertaken to deal with problems related to abuse. Although the drug problem may not be the most important problem, it is a priority that must be taken care of in some fashion before other therapies can proceed. (In the case of an abused child, of course, her or his protection from further assault must be the first priority.)

Abstinence solves SOME problems

No one should presume or pretend that abstinence simplifies or alleviates all of a drug user's difficulties. Many people in this world lead complex, chaotic lives. Some people who behave rudely or cruelly while under the influence of drugs may be only slightly less ill-behaved when drug free; they may face a lot of hard work in resolving problems with anger, depression, self-destructiveness, goal setting and perseverance. Others may find that seemingly overwhelming problems become manageable when they stop using drugs. If we were to analyze the variance of a particular trait or behavior, we might find that 40% of the variance in behavior would be related to drug use in some populations, while in others 80% could be related to drug use.

No matter how complex the situation, drug use can account for a great deal of the problem behavior and the cessation of drug use can reduce the likelihood that the behavior will occur. For instance, certain types of controlling, authoritarian, inadequate men who brutalize their wives when drunk are less likely to do so when sober. Even though the problem is not so simple that abstinence alone can solve it, abstinence from chemicals may lessen the frequency and/or severity of the abuse. It also facilitates other forms of intervention that will eliminate the abuse completely.

Action is the bottom line

Efforts to define the "real" nature of a young person's relationship with drugs are, of course, part of every assessment process, but the bottom line is to take appropriate action. What referral is best? Information about a young person and definitions of the problem are only two factors in this process. The referral options available in the community greatly influence what type of data is considered relevant and what decision is made.

The Chemical Dependency Concept

Despite the popular belief that "a teenager cannot be alcoholic," some young people do become extremely dependent on chemicals, most of them psychologically and some physically dependent as well. Whether or not the drug use is related to family, emotional or other problems, drug use for these kids takes on a life of its own. As discussed earlier, symptomatic drug use can become a primary, functionally autonomous problem. It can also progress very rapidly to addiction, especially in young males with alcoholic parents. Sometimes such young people are called chemically dependent.

An ambiguous term

The term "chemical dependency" is useful, albeit somewhat ambiguous. As a term in popular use across the country, it has helped people to avoid making an unnecessary distinction between alcohol and all other drugs. Furthermore, it also implies that a person who is dependent on one drug is chemically dependent on all drugs. Although there is some scientific basis for this theory when it is applied to drugs of the same class—e.g., those addicted to alcohol also tend to be "cross-addicted" to tranquilizers and barbiturates (Ray, 1983)—it has not been proved that dependency on one class of drugs means dependency on another class. However, anecdotal evidence abounds that people prone to abuse any drug will usually have problems with other drugs as well.

One potential difficulty with the term is that it is used to imply a construct almost identical to the disease concept of alcoholism. Just like a person with the disease of alcoholism, a chemically dependent person is presumed to have a primary, progressive and, if left untreated, fatal disease.

Didactic models

The progressive disease model is a didactic tool, not a predictive one. E. M. Jellinek, author of *The Disease Concept of Alcoholism*, developed the now well-known Jellinek Curve. It illustrates the general downward slide described by many adult male alcoholics whose moderate use of alcohol progressed to severe dependency. Dr. Vernon Johnson's description of the role of feelings in the development of chemical dependency—the Feeling Chart in his book, *I'll Quit Tomorrow*—has also proved useful in helping alcoholics and other chemically dependent people comprehend their problems and begin changing their lives.

How these models apply to any particular young drug user is a moot point, since both were derived retrospectively: In looking back over their lives, male alcoholics frequently said they experienced these progressions as the disease developed. These models tell us nothing about which of the 90% of high school students who experiment with chemicals will also go through such a process. However, the models do have a place in early-intervention programs. As didactic tools, they can serve a useful purpose in self-evaluation—allowing young people to decide for themselves how they are and are not similar to those who have become chemically dependent. For predictive purposes, however, such factors as the age of first regular use of alcohol and other drugs and the history of chemical dependency in the family are more helpful than either the Jellinek Curve or the Feeling Chart.

Some pros and cons

An emphasis on chemical dependency has both advantages and disadvantages. For the most part, prevention-oriented education and training materials on drug problems have addressed the broad range of drug use, whereas intervention-oriented materials have been based on a chemical dependency or disease model. Such an emphasis can be productive or counterproductive.

○ Focusing on the most severe problems presents the clearest model, and a clear model can be valuable for some purposes. The Jellinek Curve, for instance, offers a "governing image" that is easy to hold in the mind and thus allows drug users to assess their own behavior by comparison. For didactic purposes, then, it is superior to other, more complex sociocultural models. But, as we said earlier, models that serve a valid didactic purpose may not be valid clinical predictors of behavior.

○ If its inherent ambiguities are not understood, the chemical dependency disease model can be overemphasized and misused in program applications. In attempting to have a dramatic impact on adolescent drug users, for example, counselors should not push the idea that the progression to chronic dependency is inevitable if chemical use continues. It is not. The dangers of drug use and the possibility of addiction can be presented, however, and the model can be used as a tool for reflection and self-examination, i.e., "To what extent do I and do I not share the attributes of a chemically dependent person?"

○ Misinterpretation of the disease model may foster the erroneous assumption that any young person harmfully involved with chemicals has a primary, progressive, chronic, fatal disease. It is totally inappropriate for counselors to assess a young person using this assumption as a guiding principle.

○ There is a disadvantage in holding fast to one model. Anecdotal reports indicate that when early-intervention programs are first begun in a given area, most of the initial referrals are for heavy drug users, many of whom need immediate inpatient treatment. Some of these young people eventually come to see themselves clearly in terms of the progressive disease model of chemical dependency. This model may, therefore, be validated in the first phase of development of the early-intervention programs. However, as the programs mature, the nature of the referrals changes. The programs begin to deal with more young people whose problems with drugs and alcohol use are less severe. Overemphasis of the disease model may leave people unprepared to recognize these problems and treat them seriously.

Delusion and Denial, Very Real Factors

There is copious anecdotal evidence that delusion and denial play very important roles in the lives of those who are heavily involved with chemicals. The word "delude" is itself a wonderful term. It comes from a Latin word that means "to play, sport," and the first definition in Webster's New World Dictionary is "to fool as by false promises, wrong notions, etc.; mislead; deceive; trick."

The delusions surrounding heavy drug use generally have to do with the positive qualities people attribute to drugs, to their behavior while under the influence of drugs or to their general performance despite their use of drugs. Through many a diaphanous and tortuous twist of logic we human beings, when so motivated, are able to see pretty much what we want to see. Delusion is shored up by a great many societal supports, including popular country-western songs extolling the virtues of the honky-tonk, alcohol-saturated style of life.

The term "denial" refers to the primitive qualities of self-deception—to people's amazing ability to refuse to see the obvious negative features of their drug-related behavior. This may be because of a tremendous need to hide from pain, a desperate fear of change or concerns about getting into trouble with authorities. Coupled with outright denial are more subtle tricks of self-deception, including rationalization, minimizing and projection of blame. Compensation is another way of deceiving oneself and others. A student who can perform poorly for weeks on end in the classroom and then compensate by studying hard and passing a test may be anxious to believe that his or her drug use is not causing a problem, despite evidence to the contrary.

Like delusion, denial is also propped up by many social supports. The fear of scandal and embarrassment is often so great in families, schools and communities that instead of confronting the problem head on, people stubbornly maintain a destructive "conspiracy of silence."

To put this in perspective, it is helpful to realize that delusion and denial play a key role in *all* of life's problems, not just drug-related problems. It sometimes takes a full family meeting, attended by many relatives, to convince a family member that, as the heart specialist told him, his chest pains really are symptoms of a critical problem and warrant open-heart surgery. Similarly, some incest victims simply cannot remember the time in their lives when they were being abused because they have blocked it out of their memories.

Distortion of the concept of denial

Unfortunately in some treatment centers, schools and assessment services, any person who uses drugs is put immediately into a "damned-if-you-do, damned-if-you-don't" situation. Whenever a counselor presumes and states the presumption that a client has a particular problem in behavior or in using drugs, any denial of that presumption is interpreted as a symptom of the client's general delusion and denial regarding chemicals. This presumption of denial can be a vicious practice in treatment. It dehumanizes the client by making her or his perceptions and experiences invalid.

Denial should never be presumed. Counselors must confront, but they must confront with specific data, not with the ideology "If you are using chemicals, you will deny everything."

Not always a factor in continued use

Denial is not always a major factor in continued, harmful use of chemicals. A survey of 414 daily users of marijuana (Johnston, Bachman and O'Malley, 1982a) revealed that a surprisingly high percentage were aware of and willing to admit to having problems associated with heavy drug use. On a checklist of 15 potential problems, 43% of the users indicated that marijuana use had lowered their energy level; 37% thought it had decreased their interest in other activities; 34% thought it had hurt their school performance; 37% thought it had interfered with their ability to think clearly; and 39% thought it had damaged their relationships with their parents.

Some of those who admit to having problems may simply minimize these problems to a level that they think is acceptable. Others may, however, see the problems as serious but also may simply disregard harmful effects of drugs on their lives. These people may say, "Sure, I'm losing interest in other activities, *but* I'm no good at anything anyway" or "Well, my relationship with my parents is getting worse, *but* I wasn't getting much out of it before" or "Maybe it hurts my schoolwork, *but* schoolwork is always so boring and this is so much fun!"

To those of us working with drug users, these "buts" are crucial. Making young people aware of the deleterious effects of drugs on their lives is not always enough to prompt them to change their behavior. Knowing what makes them disregard the destruction of their health and relationships is a necessary step in helping them to lead drug-free lives.

***   ***   ***

In this chapter we reviewed some of the complex and often controversial issues that arise whenever adolescent drug use is discussed. In the next chapter we wade into the research data on adolescent drug use and consider the implications that this material has for the development of early-intervention programs.

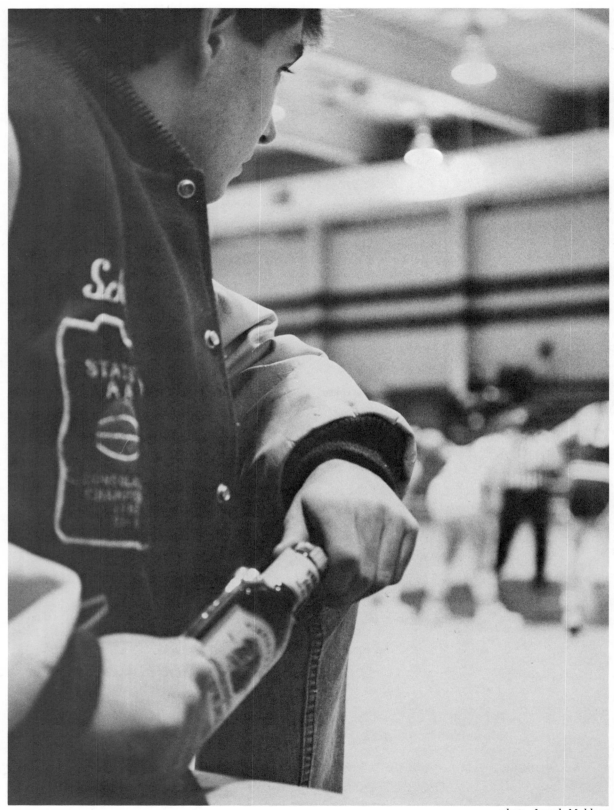

photo: Joseph Muldoon

CHAPTER THREE

THE CHALLENGE WE FACE

Trends in Drug Use

A consideration of pharmacology and statistical trends in drug use has its place in early-intervention programming. These two vast areas of knowledge can, however, absorb too much time in the planning process. In this chapter we do not cover pharmacology and statistics in depth but provide an overview and some perspectives to help distinguish the truly relevant from the merely interesting or downright boring aspects of these two topics.

The Relevance of Pharmacology

For the general purposes of program planning and development, in-depth knowledge about specific drugs and specific drug effects is not of crucial importance. How much knowledge is necessary depends on the program activity. To teach a health class on drugs, teachers must know about the physical effects of drugs. To conduct an Insight Group (described in Chapter Seven) for youths who appear to have drug problems, facilitators need to know how patterns of drug use affect emotions, self-concept, relationships and academic performance. They need such knowledge to guide discussions and stimulate self-examination. It is not at all necessary, how-

ever, to master all the street slang used to describe drug experiences. Counselors pick this up soon enough, anyway; the danger comes in using such words incorrectly. Knowledge gained from working with young drug users will soon surpass all book learning.

For most purposes, then, a shelf of reliable reference materials suffices. Turn to them when questions about drugs and drug effects arise. The books described in "Recommended Reading on Drugs and Drug Effects" on page 32 should be sufficient to answer most technical questions about drugs.

One issue that deserves close attention and that is not frequently discussed is the reluctance of adults to accept, without reservation, the fact that alcohol is a psychoactive drug. This issue has direct relevance to the planning and development of early-intervention programs.

Alcohol is a drug

Popular opinion notwithstanding, alcohol is and always has been the leading drug of use and abuse in the United States. Alcohol is not "like a drug" or "almost a drug in the way people react to it." It *is* a drug, like all other mood-altering chemicals. Ethyl alcohol is the psychoactive component of alcoholic bever-

Recommended Reading on Drugs and Drug Effects

Steering Clear: Helping Your Child Through the High-Risk Drug Years
By Dorothy Cretcher. Minneapolis: Winston Press, Inc., 1982, 112 pages.

Although this book is written expressly for parents, it is appropriate for anyone working with adolescents. Drawing on previous research, her own survey of treatment and prevention agencies and her interviews with adults and adolescents, Cretcher assesses the nature of and problems related to the most commonly used drugs in the United States. She also offers suggestions to help guide parent-child discussions about drugs and urges cooperation, rather than conflict, between parents and schools.

Drugs, Society, & Human Behavior
By Oakley Ray, Ph.D.
St. Louis: The C. V. Mosby Company, 1983, 512 pages.

For those who want to delve deeper, but not get lost in a surfeit of superfluous facts, Oakley Ray's book is the next best source. Although it contains too much information to be absorbed in a single reading, *Drugs, Society, & Human Behavior* is a valuable introduction to many topics relevant to drug use. In the first three chapters of this book, Dr. Ray presents an overview of the crucial issues related to drug use and reviews the history of drug regulation in the United States. Chapter Four contains a summary of the issues and research on the relationships between drug use and driving, crimes, violence, sports, sexual behavior, pregnancy and bad LSD trips. Chapters Five through Nineteen cover the basics of the physiology and pharmacology of drug effects as well as a chapter-by-chapter consideration of each of the major categories of drugs.

Mystification and Drug Misuse
By Henry L. Lennard, Leon J. Epstein, Arnold Bernstein and Donald C. Ransom. San Francisco: Jossey-Bass, Inc., 1971, 139 pages.

The perspective of the authors is made clear in their introduction:

"Although most of the current voluminous writing about the misuse of drugs concerns the misuse of psychoactive agents by young people, and especially the use of drugs obtained illegally, we feel that to decry the use and misuse of drugs by young people while paying so little attention to the growing use and misuse of psychoactive agents in general, both those prescribed by physicians and those obtained over the counter without prescription, is highly misleading and unproductive."

This book in no way condones drug use by young people, but it puts adolescent drug use into a helpful perspective. This book can be useful in diffusing the self-righteousness that colors so many discussions by adults about teenage drug abuse. At the time of this writing, *Mystification and Drug Misuse* was no longer being printed. However, copies can still be obtained from many libraries or the bookshelves of interested professionals.

ages. It is a general depressant of the central nervous system and is very capable of producing psychological and physical dependence. "Alcohol Abuse: Our Number One Drug Problem" on page 34 explains why alcohol abuse has maintained its position as the greatest threat to the well-being of our young people.

Why do people make a distinction between alcohol and other drugs? This is a complex question. Certainly, alcohol has different effects than some other drugs. However, if pharmacology alone were the basis for separating alcohol from other drugs, then minor tranquilizers and barbiturates should also be separated from other drugs because they have effects similar to those of alcohol. People are reluctant to consider alcohol a drug for many reasons. Although none of the following reasons fit all people, more than one usually applies when the alcohol/drug dichotomy is argued:

- *The known vs. the unknown*. People think they are familiar with how bad alcohol can be and are not afraid of what widespread alcohol use will do to society. Although many admit that alcohol abuse causes problems, they feel they are aware of just how bad the problems are and are not worried that things will get worse. Less is known, in general, about other drugs, and some fear that a disaster of unprecedented proportions awaits us. These people do not realize that the disaster is here. The slaughter of people on our highways by drunken drivers causes more loss and grief than the use of any other drug does. Family problems, domestic violence and child abuse related to alcoholism are major problems that are just coming to the attention of the general public.

- *Our national drug of choice*. Alcohol is the drug of choice for many people. Many of those involved in community mobilization for drug problems attend gatherings where parents and community leaders meet to consider problems and solutions to "the drug problem." At some of those gatherings, cocktails are served, even to people who obviously

have trouble with their alcohol use. In a great many ways we tend to unconsciously accept as normal the harmful effects of alcohol.

- *The bureaucratic imperative*. Vast bureaucracies have grown up to deal with drugs and alcohol as though they were separate problems. There is a major government agency for alcohol problems, the National Institute on Alcoholism and Alcohol Abuse (NIAAA), and one for drug problems, the National Institute on Drug Abuse (NIDA). Although at the time of this writing it appears that these two agencies may eventually be combined, their separation has affected not only practical approaches to problems but also has often caused researchers to make basic presumptions before doing research. Some very expensive studies, for instance, have been conducted to define various patterns of drug abuse without including assessments of alcohol use. We may learn, then, that use of tranquilizers by women drops off at a certain age, but we do not know whether or not this corresponds to an increase in alcohol use. In many ways, on the state and national level, the literature published by these two agencies has contributed to the arbitrary separation of drugs from alcohol. The Law Enforcement Assistance Administration has contributed to the confusion by pumping out literature and training packets on "illegal" drugs that carry no mention of the illegal use of alcohol.

- *Trying to become experts on one drug*. We have heard it said by people in anti-drug groups that they are focusing on marijuana because they do not want to spread themselves too thin. They want to become experts on at least one drug so that they can really educate today's youth and set up truly effective programs for that one drug. Making people aware of the deleterious effects of marijuana has been useful in encouraging people to stop using the drug. It can also be one way to motivate communities to become interested in developing a drug program. However, it is senseless to offer help to marijuana users and not offer help to users of alcohol. Most heavy users of marijuana also use

Alcohol Abuse: Our Number One Drug Problem

There was an interesting study conducted during the 1960s (McKinney, 1966) in which alcohol was compared to marijuana, stimulants, sedatives, opiates, caffeine and nicotine. The author was attempting to determine which drug was most likely to cause addiction in the average American. Factors considered were: ability to addict (physically and psychologically), simplicity of use, simplicity of manufacture and societal supports. Alcohol won, hands down, the title of "ideally addicting drug."

A simple, common sense review of the attributes of alcohol and alcohol use in this country would probably lead most of us to the same conclusion. Consider the following aspects of alcohol:

o *Legality.* Alcohol is legal. Everyone of drinking age can buy it and most people under age have no trouble purchasing it either.

o *Acceptability.* Alcohol is socially acceptable among young people and even among many of their parents. Every coffee table in the country has a magazine with an ad of a beautifully photographed cocktail party with beautiful people sitting in beautiful leather chairs drinking beside their beautiful fireplaces. Compare these ads with the rag-enshrouded skeletons holding needles in their boney fists that are used to symbolize drug abuse.

o *Social tolerance.* Even the abuse of alcohol is usually tolerated and frequently condoned. Law enforcement people might look the other way for a little drunken rowdiness but become shocked and angered by a young person who is high on marijuana or having a bad LSD trip.

o *Reliability.* Alcohol is a reliable drug for most people. Its results are predictable. The fact that many other drugs are somewhat unpredictable for some people—and thus more dangerous in terms of the possibility of overdoses—has been cited as proof that they are "worse" than alcohol. However, as a contributing factor to addiction, alcohol's consistently satisfying effects are among its most seductive features.

o *Slow development of problems.* Alcohol addiction develops slowly for most people. It seems to happen almost imperceptibly over a ten- to twelve-year period, although with younger people it seems to progress more rapidly. It is often so gradual that those addicted, even the most severely addicted, actually do not know what has happened to them. They have their low periods, but they recover temporarily and are thus deceived.

o *Many styles of abuse.* There are many styles of alcohol abuse. Some people simply get obnoxious when they are drunk; some thoroughly embarrass themselves or others; some drive wildly; and some are more reserved. Some groups in our culture only notice one type of drug abuse and are oblivious to other types.

o *Enabling.* Many people are willing to cover up for the problem drinker. Problem drinkers frequently establish relationships with people who enable them to keep drinking: the wife who makes excuses to the boss; the friend who always agrees to have a drink or two with a person who doesn't want to drink alone; the supervisor who tries to help the employee out by assigning easy jobs when he or she is hungover.

While other drugs manifest some of these attributes, alcohol is the only one that combines them all.

alcohol. Drug problems can hardly be addressed if alcohol problems are not addressed as well.

■ *A lack of assertiveness with our children.* There is a certain lack of assertiveness among parents who are confused about the position they would be in if they were to admit that alcohol is a drug as dangerous as marijuana. They may be attempting to justify their use of alcohol by saying that it is intrinsically less dangerous. Once alcohol is also labeled a drug, however, parents have to take a different stand. They have to say that although they do use alcohol, they realize that it is something that should not be done without some consideration of possible consequences. A certain amount of maturity is needed before one can use alcohol properly, and the use of *any* mood-altering chemical must be avoided while a person is engaged in the basic developmental tasks of adolescence. We must admit that we *are* taking risks when we use alcohol, but assessment of those risks requires a level of maturity and experience not available to most adolescents.

■ *The alcohol problems of adults.* Many adults are unable to use alcohol properly. Some are our friends, some are school principals, some are working with us on anti-drug campaigns. For this reason it is often more comfortable to avoid the issue of alcohol problems—comfortable for a time, that is, but harmful to programs in the long run.

■ *"If we admit that alcohol is as dangerous as marijuana, then we'd have to legalize marijuana."* Well, luckily, it is not that simple. Whether or not we should throw another powerful drug into the mass market is an issue that takes in far, far more than the relative dangerousness of the drug in question. There is no likelihood at all that marijuana will be legalized in the near future, no matter how honest we are about the effects of alcohol.

■ *Alcoholics Anonymous.* Alcoholics Anonymous (AA) has long been the single most effective way of helping adult alcoholics stay sober. It has saved literally thousands, per-

haps millions, of lives and saved years of suffering for families. It has also been a powerful political force. People espousing the AA philosophy have had a tremendous impact on the way services for alcohol problems have developed in this country. In the 1950s, a consensus developed in the AA fellowship that AA should not be open to people who had problems primarily with drugs other than alcohol. This may well have been a wise decision for AA and for people who voluntarily join the fellowship. Joining AA is a personal choice that one makes about one's own life. Schools, courts and social service agencies, however, must serve a broad clientele and do not have the prerogative of either excluding people with drug problems or working only with non-alcohol-related problems. Furthermore, what may have been helpful for AA in the 1950s may no longer be practical. A survey conducted by AA of its membership indicated that increasingly greater numbers of its membership have polydrug addictions (Alcoholics Anonymous, 1981).

There are probably many more reasons people have for separating alcohol from other drugs. It is sometimes appropriate to study the different effects of and interrelationships among drugs and groups of drugs, but it is not appropriate to make the *a priori* assumption that alcohol should be in one category and all other mood-altering chemicals in another.

Please note that we are not saying that all drugs are alike and that there need be no distinction made between them. We *are* saying that some distinctions are artificial and unproductive, and that some lack of distinction has been harmful. Alcohol should not be separated from all other drugs. On the other hand, marijuana should not be classified as a narcotic, as it has been by many law enforcement agencies.

For purposes of early intervention for drug problems, programs must be set up to deal with any drug. If not, the community is left with a program that may eliminate or limit the use of one drug, while young people simply shift their interests to other drugs. People may learn a lot about alcohol or learn a lot about marijuana without learning about how closely interrelated the two drugs are.

Trends in Drug Use

There is no dearth of statistics regarding drug and alcohol use. Just as people developing social services have been accused of trying to solve problems by throwing money at them, some government agencies have apparently hoped to solve drug and alcohol problems by throwing statistics at them. As a way of portraying the length and breadth of the suffering caused by drug and alcohol abuse, statistical summaries are but pale reflections of real life. Nonetheless, in the day-to-day struggle against drug use and dependency problems, it is easy for beleaguered combatants to lose perspective. Sometimes statistical summaries can help in this regard.

This section has two purposes. First, it provides a useful overview of the impact of drug use on our society. Second, it serves as a resource for the statistical backup needed to write proposals or articles for local publications or to provide inservice training for staff members. The best way to approach this material is to read it over quickly for the general concepts that the data represent and to refer back to specific references when the need arises.

A note of caution. Although the statistics cited in this chapter cover much of the material available through early 1985, trends will change and this will no longer be the most current resource. The material is, however, illustrative of many issues that will continue to be germane well into the next decade. Furthermore, since each statistical area covered also includes comments on the relevance of the data to program planning, readers should be able to gain some understanding of how to integrate new findings into the model presented in this book.

Rather than providing a comprehensive survey of the literature (many surveys are available in a variety of journals), we present a number of general statements that we feel are supported by the literature. We cite some corroborating studies and offer subjective comments concerning the relevance of these facts to early-intervention programming.

Teenage alcohol and marijuana use is very common

According to findings from a nationwide study (Johnston, O'Malley and Bachman, 1984), 92.6% of high school seniors had tried alcohol, 87.3% had used it in the previous year, 69.4% had used alcohol during the previous month and 5.5% admitted daily use (Figure 3-1). Forty-one percent stated that on at least one occasion during the prior two-week period they had had five or more consecutive drinks. In terms of marijuana use, 57% had tried it, 42.3% had used the drug during the previous year, 27% had used it during the previous month and 5.5% admitted daily use (Figure 3-2).

Relevance to programming

Drug use has become so prevalent that, in and of itself, it tells us very little about a particular young person. Given the fact that more than 90% of our high school seniors have tried alcohol and almost 60% have tried marijuana, it should be obvious that many different types of students with many different kinds of problems and strengths are using drugs to some extent. No single form of intervention is likely to work for all of them. Furthermore, a single incident of drug use, without further information, may tell us almost nothing about the young person and what should be done to curb his or her drug use. When an incident of drug use comes to light, further investigation is necessary to determine the extent of the problem.

If parents, schools and communities can begin to reassert their legitimate expectation that young people remain drug free, the work of early-intervention programs will be easier. Many casual experimenters will cease doing drugs when it is clear that their families,

Figure 3-1 Alcohol Use by High School Students

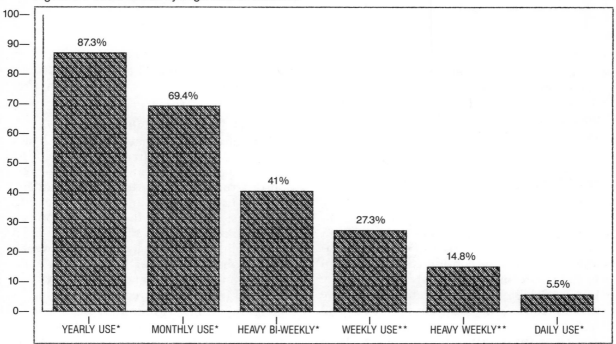

Figure 3-1.   Although the two studies from which these numbers were derived used slightly different research methods, this graphic integration of their findings gives a good overall picture of adolescent alcohol use (Johnston, Bachman and O'Malley*, 1984, studied high school seniors in the class of 1983; Lowman**, 1981, studied 10th through 12th graders).

Figure 3-2 Marijuana Use by High School Students

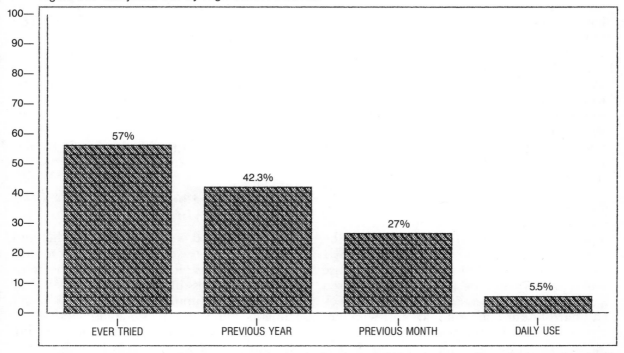

Figure 3-2.   Almost a third of the high school seniors in the class of 1983 had used marijuana in the previous month (Johnston, O'Malley and Bachman, 1984).

schools, law enforcement agencies, employers and others expect it. Those young people who are willing to risk various sanctions to continue using drugs will be a smaller group and a group in greater need of direct services.

Studies of heavy drug use describe clear targets for early intervention

A closer look at the statistics in Figure 3-1 reveals that there is a clear target group in immediate need of intervention. Looking at Figure 3-1, we can see that 5.5% of the students studied can be considered daily users of alcohol (Johnston et al., 1984) and 14.8% are "heavy weekly users" (Lowman, 1981). There will, of course, be variations at the local level.

In their study of a cross section of inner-city, urban and suburban schools, Cooper, Olson and Fournier (1977) found that 22% of the students were "frequent users," i.e., they used *at least* one drug four or more times per week. Pandina, White and Yorke (1981) reported that 10.3% of the students in a high school population were "very high users," with an average Substance Use Index (SUI) score of 70.2.

The SUI is a complex, statistically derived scale in which many different patterns of drug use can, if they are judged to cause problems of a similar degree of severity, receive similar scores. For example, a student who used marijuana daily, beer several times per week and hard liquor and barbiturates once a month and who had experimented with but was not currently using amphetamines, hallucinogens and cocaine would receive an SUI(f) score of 70.09 for frequency of substance use. (Other factors that must be taken into account to calculate a total SUI score are the recency of use and extent of use over a person's lifetime.) A student who used marijuana daily, beer several times per week and hard liquor once a month and who had experimented with but was not currently using amphetamines and hallucinogens would receive an SUI(f) score of 60.2 for frequency of substance use. Pandina and associ-

ates (1981) found that 15.6% of the students studied were "high users," with an average SUI score of 59.57.

Relevance to programming

We can safely assume that daily use or heavy weekly use of mood-altering chemicals requires some intervention by early-intervention program services. Although *all* students who are using alcohol and other drugs illegally must (or should) face the appropriate consequences of their actions, there is likely to be a solid group of daily and heavy weekly users, probably between 15% and 25% depending on the school and community, who will need immediate direct intervention.

This is the bare minimum, of course. A great number of students with slightly less severe drug problems will also come to light and merit assistance. Furthermore, even if heavy weekly alcohol users or daily marijuana users are not currently experiencing apparent consequences—and most probably are—it is likely that most will have serious problems at some time in their lives if they do not get help while they are still in school. The binge-drinking group, the 40% to 50% of students who tend to drink heavily at least once every two weeks, will also merit close attention. The majority probably will not be lifelong problem drinkers. However, this volatile and dangerous drinking pattern is responsible for innumerable highway accidents and should be a critical target for all prevention and intervention programs.

Alcohol and marijuana top the list of mood-altering substances

When compared with the use of alcohol and marijuana, the use of other drugs is considerably less (Johnston et al., 1984). The most widely used class of illegal drugs other than marijuana is stimulants, with 26.9% of all students admitting to some use and 8.9% having used stimulants at least once during the past 30 days. As shown in Figure 3-3, 0.8% of all students admitted to using stimulants on a daily basis.

Relevance to programming

Unlike alcohol and marijuana, other drugs wax and wane in popularity. It is important that early-intervention programs do not become too invested in combating the use of one drug or base their very reason for existence on the dangers posed by any one type of drug, such as PCP, amphetamines or cocaine.

The rate of alcohol use has been stable

According to an analysis of the 1975-1983 trends in drug use among high school students (Johnston et al., 1984), daily marijuana use has dropped by almost half since 1978 (from 10.7% to 5.5%) and annual use has decreased from 50.8% to 42.3% since 1979. The incidence of alcohol use, including that of daily use, which has hovered around 6% since 1975, has been more stable. The incidence of occasional binge drinking, i.e., having five or more consecutive drinks at least once during the prior two-week period, has also remained steady at 41% since 1979.

Relevance to programming

The relatively stable use of alcohol indicates that it is more deeply ingrained in our society. In addition to showing less variation over time, alcohol use shows less variation across geographical regions. The incidence of lifetime marijuana use among teenagers is 11.3% lower in rural areas (54.6%) than in large metropolitan areas (65.9%). The incidence of alcohol use among adolescents is only 3% lower in rural areas (91.3%) compared to large metropolitan areas (94.5%) (Johnston, Bachman and O'Malley, 1982a). While there are more guidelines in our society for regular, non-problem-causing use of alcohol than for marijuana use, there is also a great deal of support for alcohol abuse. When the drug alcohol is considered part of the drug problem, the elimination of drug abuse among teenagers is still a very long way off.

Daily drug use is generally twice as high among boys than among girls

According to findings from a nationwide study (Johnston et al., 1984), daily use of marijuana was more than twice as high among male students (7.3%) as among female students (3.2%). Likewise, daily use of alcohol was more than twice as high among male students (7.7%) as among female students (2.8%). Also, male students tended to do more binge drinking than female students (50% vs. 31%).

Relevance to programming

Although male and female high school students do not differ greatly in terms of their degree of lifetime use of alcohol or marijuana, the difference between the two sexes regarding daily use is clear. It would not be unusual, then, for more male than female students to be brought into an early-intervention program for problems related to their own drug use.

The more alcohol adolescents drink, the more likely they are to use other drugs

In "Facts for Planning, No. 2: Alcohol Use As an Indicator of Psychoactive Drug Use Among the Nation's Senior High School Students" (1981-1982) Lowman presented some interesting data concerning psychoactive drug use among alcohol users. Figure 3-4 shows how lifetime experience with marijuana use varies with different patterns of alcohol use among teenagers. Lowman derived the following additional conclusions from her research:

- *Most marijuana users are also alcohol users.* Only 6% of high school students who used marijuana in the year prior to the survey reported that they abstained from alcohol.

- *Marijuana use increases in extent and frequency among high school students who are heavier users of alcohol.* An estimated 63% of heavy drinkers had used marijuana *within the previous month*, compared with only 4%

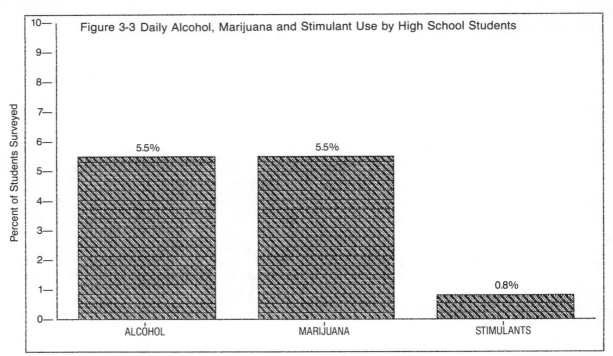

Figure 3-3. Daily use of alcohol and marijuana is almost seven times as prevalent as the daily use of stimulants (Johnston, O'Malley and Bachman, 1984).

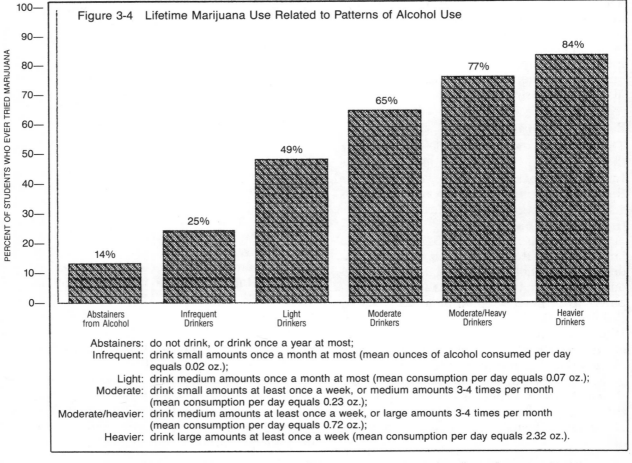

Figure 3-4. The more adolescents drink, the more likely they are to have tried marijuana (Lowman, 1981-82).

of alcohol abstainers, 9% of infrequent drinkers, 21% of light drinkers, 36% of moderate drinkers and 53% of moderate to heavy drinkers.

- *Use of seven types of psychoactive drugs other than alcohol and marijuana is more extensive and more frequent among high school students who are heavy users of alcohol.* An estimated 16% of high school students who are heavy drinkers had used stimulants during the previous month, in contrast to 1% of the students who are infrequent drinkers. An estimated 10% of the heavy drinkers had used cocaine during the same one-month period, in contrast to 0.3% of the infrequent drinkers.

- *Polydrug use—the use of two or more psychoactive drugs other than alcohol—is more extensive and more frequent among high school students who drink more heavily.* The same strong association found between drinking levels and marijuana use also occurs between drinking levels and polydrug use. Forty-six percent of the heavy drinkers said that at some time they had used two or more psycho-active drugs other than alcohol, compared with 5% of the infrequent drinkers. During the month preceding the survey, 24% of heavy drinkers had used two or more types of psychoactive drugs other than alcohol, whereas only 1% of the infrequent drinkers had.

Relevance to programming

Some alcohol treatment professionals are not competent in other areas of drug abuse and some drug treatment professionals are not competent when it comes to dealing with alcohol-related problems. Early-intervention programs need professionals competent in both areas. The dichotomy between drugs and alcohol is dysfunctional no matter who the client is, but it is especially so when applied to adolescents in an early-intervention setting.

Almost one third of students report serious consequences related to alcohol use

In "Facts for Planning, No. 4: Alcohol Misuse by Adolescents" (1982), Rachal and associates described the extent of negative consequences related to alcohol use. They found that 31.2% of the senior high school students surveyed in 1978 were "alcohol misusers," i.e., they "reported drunkenness at least six times in the past year or reported negative consequences two or more times during the year in at least three of five areas considered." Sixty-nine percent of the misusers were so classified because of frequent drunkenness, but this does not mean that they avoided other harmful consequences. Figure 3-5 shows the proportion of alcohol misusers who experienced other consequences as well.

Relevance to programming

Bear in mind that the use of additional drugs can only add to the 31.2% of students who definitely experienced negative consequences related to alcohol use.

Chemical dependency is not the only drug problem

To quote the pamphlet "Alcohol and Youth" (1980) published by NIAAA:

> Alcohol misuse or problem drinking among adolescents is more often associated with episodic, heavy drinking than with alcoholism (Smart, 1979). Teenage problem drinkers usually do not suffer from physical disabilities (such as liver damage) associated with alcoholism, but they do experience other severe, acute consequences (Donovan and Jessor, 1978; Rachal, et al., 1980). While driving under the influence of alcohol, they can be involved in fatal or otherwise serious traffic accidents. They can get into trouble with the police, school authorities and teachers. Drinking can interfere with their schoolwork, their relationships with dates or friends, and their ability to communicate with their families (Donovan and Jessor, 1978; Mayer and Filstead, 1979; and Rachal et al., 1980).

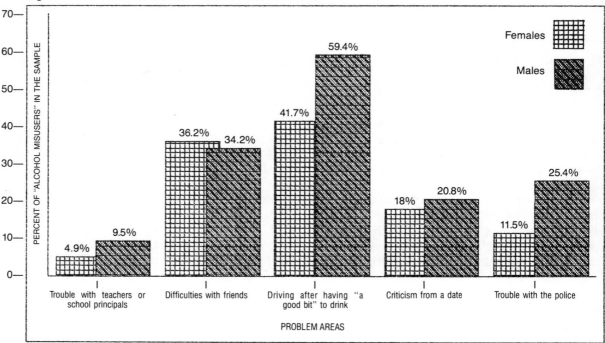

Figure 3-5 Problems Related to the Misuse of Alcohol

Figure 3-5. Numbers represent the percentage of "alcohol misusers" in the sample who reported at least one occurrence of alcohol-related trouble during the past year (Rachal, Guess, Hubbard and Maisto, 1982).

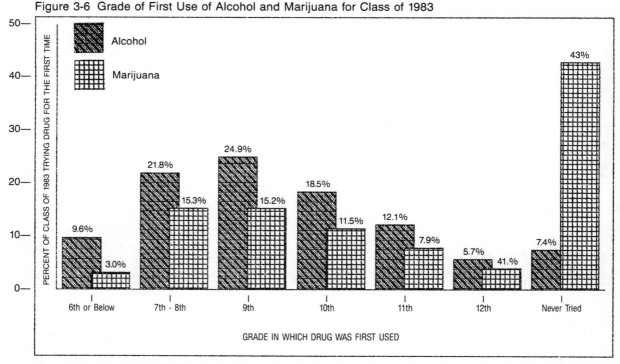

Figure 3-6 Grade of First Use of Alcohol and Marijuana for Class of 1983

Figure 3-6. More than half of the students tested had tried alcohol and more than a third had tried marijuana by the time they left ninth grade (Johnston, O'Malley, and Bachman 1984).

This theme is echoed in the National Council on Alcoholism's pamphlet "Aspects of Youthful Drinking" (1979) where, after summarizing a wide range of data, O'Gorman and Lacks concluded that adolescents are more prone to develop acute problems than chronic problems related to alcohol use.

Relevance to programming

The researchers cited above corroborate the statements made in Chapter Two concerning the progression of chemical dependency. Many services for adolescent alcohol problems use an adult model in which alcoholism is described as a "primary, progressive, chronic and fatal disease." While some adolescents are already or are likely to become alcoholic in this sense, it is very difficult to tell which ones will and which ones will not. Consultants who make the presumption, explicitly or implicitly, that young, problem drinkers are alcoholic or chemically dependent should not be used in early-intervention programs. This also holds for written and audiovisual materials that espouse the same presumption.

Experimentation picks up markedly after sixth grade

Of the seniors graduating from high school in l983, 3.0% had tried marijuana and 9.6% had tried alcohol before the seventh grade (Johnston et al., 1984). In the next three years, experimentation increased tremendously. By the end of ninth grade, 56.6% of the whole class had tried alcohol and 33.5% had tried marijuana (Figure 3-6). This means that 60.7% of those who used alcohol and 58.9% of those who used marijuana during their high school years had tried these drugs by the end of the ninth grade.

Relevance to programming

In many, but not all communities, the major focus of programming before the seventh grade is children suffering from their parents' drinking, not intervention for personal drug use. Some schools and agencies have adjusted their prevention and intervention efforts to provide special programs for young people in the sixth and seventh grades to prepare them for dealing with the expected increase in pressure to use drugs during the eighth and ninth grades. Again, local trends may vary considerably; some school districts report a significant amount of drug use in the fifth grade or earlier.

The pressure to try drugs and alcohol begins before the sixth grade

The classroom publication, *Weekly Reader*, polled students in grades four through twelve about drugs and alcohol (Borton, 1983). A sample from the 100,000 students responding to the poll was selected, analyzed and weighted to adjust for the U.S. population distribution. The findings indicated that as early as fourth grade about 35% of students felt there was "some" to "a lot" of pressure from peers to try alcohol and 29% felt there was pressure to try marijuana. The motivation for trying drugs and liquor in the lower grades appeared to be the desire to "feel older."

Relevance to programming

This finding recalls the "trickle down effect" discussed in Chapter Two. Although there is a big difference between "feeling peer pressure" and actually doing drugs, program planners had better be prepared to deal with fourth grade drug users. Since services for dealing with such a problem have not been well conceptualized or developed, the tendency may be to ignore such behavior. Early-intervention programs will sometimes have to deal with very young drug users, and in some school districts they may have to do so on a regular basis.

One fifth of high school students have a family member who has received drug counseling or treatment

In a survey of 11,000 students in Minnesota (Benson et al., 1983), 23% of all twelfth graders indicated that some member of their family had a problem with alcohol or other drugs at the time of the survey and 20% indicated that a family member had had professional counseling or treatment for chemical abuse or dependency. This finding is similar to that reported by Woodson (1976), who found that 16% to 23% of a sample of college students had an alcoholic parent.

Relevance to programming

Given these findings, it would be appropriate to offer such services as concerned persons groups to students who are being adversely affected by the drinking or drug use of a relative or friend. Because the specific population of drug users has an even higher incidence of alcoholism among family members, any program offering services to drug users should be prepared to deal with the issue of parental alcoholism. This does not mean that people working in early-intervention programs must always perform direct interventions with parents or be involved in any counseling with parents. If school personnel, court officials and social service professionals are aware of the resources in their communities for supporting children from troubled families and for working with those families, they should make the families aware of these resources. Chapters Seven and Eight contain some suggestions for working with the children of alcoholics and their parents.

Medical and drug services will find a high incidence of parental alcoholism

Young people with medical and/or behavioral problems appear to be more likely to have a parent who is alcoholic or has a drinking problem. According to Biek (1981), 57% of the young people visiting a teen clinic for medical treatment or to see a social worker had a parent with a drinking problem. Also, they had 47% more somatic complaints than the young people who did not have a parent with a drinking problem.

In studying the clients of an inner-city pediatric clinic, Bosma and Jensen (1976) found that more than 50% of the children aged 2 to 18 who were referred because of behavioral disorders had an alcoholic parent. In addition, 82% of 128 male adolescents on probation and 67% of 200 adolescents referred for help with problems related to drugs had an alcoholic parent.

In a study of 505 children and adolescents who were admitted to a hospital emergency room for attempted suicide, researchers found that more than half had family members suffering from "psychiatric illness" (Garfinkel, Froese and Hood, 1982). They found that "among the members of their families who had psychiatric illnesses, drug abuse/alcoholism predominated (32.6% of the mothers, 59.1% of the fathers and 24.2% of the siblings)."

Relevance to programming

While the general student population certainly has its share of young people who are adversely affected by parental drinking problems, the rate can be much higher among certain subgroups. Medical and court settings can be very important places for identifying and assisting the children of alcoholics.

The children of alcoholics face a high risk of having drug problems

The evidence is irrefutable. The children of alcoholics run a higher-than-average risk of becoming alcoholics themselves or at least of having severe problems related to chemicals. Vaillant and Milofsky (1982) conducted a 33-year follow-up study of about 400 men who had served as the nondelinquent controls in a longitudinal study of delinquency. In their effort to discover which of several possible predictors of adult alcoholism had been present in these people's youth, the authors found two important factors, heredity and ethnicity. Men with several alcoholic relatives were three times as likely to become dependent on alcohol as those with no alcoholic relatives. In addition, the Irish were seven times more likely to be alcohol dependent than descendants of Mediterranean ethnic groups (Italian, Jewish, Greek, Portuguese and Syrian), and those of Northern European descent were six times as likely to be alcohol dependent. In *The New Drinkers* (1980), Reginald Smart cites a number of studies showing that the rates of alcoholism among the parents of those diagnosed alcoholic range from 50% to 60%.

In a study of seventh and eighth graders in Minnesota (Namakkal and Mangen, 1979), students with family members who had been through treatment programs for alcoholism or drug abuse reported significantly greater personal use of all illicit substances examined (Figure 3-7). Overall, 17.2% of students reported that a family member had undergone treatment for alcoholism. Of that group, 24.9% reported current marijuana use of at least twice weekly, compared with 14.7% of the other students. The incidence of daily use of hard liquor for students with parents who had completed treatment was 4.1%, compared with 1.6% for the rest of the students. Furthermore, 28.7% of the students with parents who had drinking problems reported using hard liquor at least once a week, compared with 18.1% of other students.

Relevance to programming

Clearly, the children of alcoholics deserve an early-intervention service to help them become aware of their risk and to help them cope with the problems of living in a home that may still be feeling the acute effects of alcohol problems. Everyone accepts it as a given that peer pressure has a great impact on adolescent chemical use. We are also realizing that parental characteristics have a great deal to do with the amount of alcohol use among students. Both prevention and intervention programs should involve parents on a variety of levels. Parents must realize that alcohol is a drug just like any other drug and that their own drinking behavior may influence their children's drug use.

Many heavy drug users have been victims of child abuse

According to Rosenker's unpublished study (1982) of 261 drug abusing adolescents referred for treatment at the Chanhassen Adolescent Evaluation Unit in Chanhassen, Minnesota, 57% of the girls and 8% of the boys were victims of incest. In another Minnesota study (Omegon, Inc., 1983), 73% of all residents of a long-term residential treatment center for adolescent drug abusers were found to be victims of previously unreported physical and sexual abuse. Sullivan (1980) conducted a study of the adult clients of a long-term residential program for people with severe drug problems and histories of criminal behavior. She found that 68% of the clients had been physically abused as children; 41% (86% of the women, 28% of the men) had been sexually abused; 78% had been subjected to emotional abuse; and 56% had been neglected.

Relevance to programming

The intertwining of the issues of child abuse and adolescent drug abuse is a matter of serious concern to all of us who work with young people. Certainly, not every drug user has been a victim of abuse, but a significant number have, and it is important that these young victims' drug abuse and other negative behaviors not be the sole focus of all interventions. When a person is viewed primarily as a "drug user" or "incorrigible," most of his or her problems are attributed to those characteristics. Other important issues are often ignored.

The number of risk factors is predictive of heavy drug use

The task of reading studies on the psychosocial correlates of drug use is often disheartening. While any particular study may appear to be thorough, valid and meticulously implemented, the conclusions of two or more studies can be contradictory at worst or disparate at the least. One study may find that low self-esteem and dependent personality traits are related to drug abuse, while another study may find that independence and self-assurance are also related to drug use.

The study by Rutgers University researchers (Bry, McKeon and Pandina, 1982) offers hope for those of us searching for coherence amid the chaos. Instead of trying to determine how specific individual factors or specific combinations of factors are related to

the seriousness of a young person's problem with chemicals, they tested the hypothesis that the mere number of risk factors in a person's life is predictive of the extent of drug use. They worked with a sample of 1,960 high school students. The six risk factors considered were low grades (Ds and Fs); independent use of alcohol (outside of the family) before age 13; lack of religious affiliation; psychological distress; low self-esteem; and problems with perceptions of parental love. Confirming the hypothesis, results showed that students exhibiting *four* of these risk factors were 4.5 times more likely to be involved in "very heavy drug use" than the general population of high school students.

Relevance to programming

Factors related to drug use are not necessarily causal factors, i.e., problems with grades and

Figure 3-7 Alcohol and Marijuana Use Related to Parental Drug Abuse

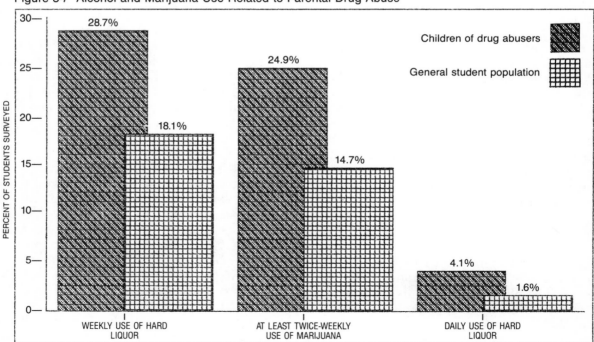

Figure 3-7.   A Minnesota study found markedly higher levels of alcohol and marijuana use by the children of alcoholics/drug abusers than in the general student population (Namakkal and Mangen, 1979).

with parents do not necessarily cause drug use. It may well be that drug use is causing other problems or exacerbating preexisting problems. This is an important distinction. A young person whose grades have dropped from As to Cs or Ds in the two years since he began using drugs heavily may be treated differently than a consistently marginal achiever whose grades dropped from Ds to Fs at the onset of drug use. Rather than helping us predict who, in the future, will become heavily involved in drugs, this type of information can help us assess who at present is likely to be heavily involved with chemicals. If a student has been caught using marijuana on the school grounds and she or he is having a lot of difficulty in school, possesses a poor self-concept and has a poor relationship with her or his parents, the likelihood of a serious drug problem increases. Care must be taken, however, to keep staff members from presuming that no drug problem worthy of intervention is present unless problems with school, courts or self-esteem are apparent.

***   ***   ***

The major point to be drawn from this chapter is that "drug problems" cannot be described with broad, ideologically based models. We must adjust our programs so that they can handle the tremendous variation among drug users regarding the degree of their involvement with chemicals and the extent to which other problems are related to their drug use. In the next chapter we begin looking at the need for a protracted, incremental intervention process and see how it fits into some social service systems.

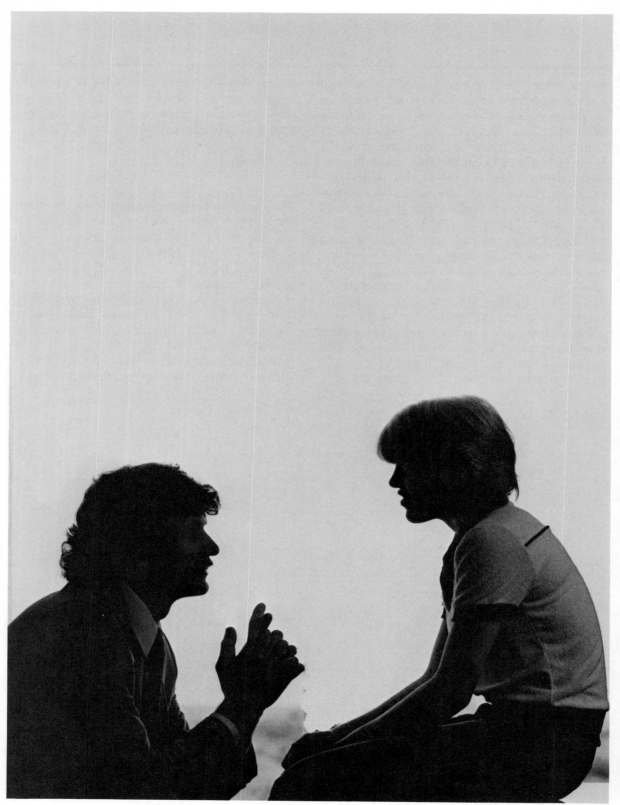

photo: Jeffrey Grosscup

CHAPTER FOUR

A FLEXIBLE MODEL

Make the Action Fit the Need

The success of early-intervention programs depends on both obvious and subtle factors. It depends on how well adults recognize and react to the problem behavior of adolescents; how open adults are to hearing the concerns that young people want to share; how much young people trust the adults around them; how much adults within an agency and throughout the community trust one another; and how prepared service providers are to deal with a range of drug use and related problems.

The success of early-intervention programs also depends on the involvement of and cooperation among educational, social service, law enforcement and judicial systems in the community. The need for such interaction is twofold: First, these systems tend to reach different segments of the younger population. If the adults in one of these key systems do not respond appropriately to troubled young people, those youths may not seek or be offered help until the problem reaches crisis proportions. Second, cooperation, or the lack of it, among these systems could mean the difference between a young person receiving real help or being lost in a bureaucratic shuffle.

In this chapter we consider some of the advantages and disadvantages of the juvenile justice and social service systems in providing early-intervention services. To understand how these systems or components of these systems can work together in the early-intervention process, we must understand the concept of incremental intervention.

Incremental Intervention

How various systems work with a young drug user is determined to a great extent by what has or has not already been tried in his or her case. Incremental intervention is a way to intervene with adolescents in a manner appropriate to their needs.

There is a form of structured intervention, usually used with adults, that involves family members and friends of an identified alcoholic in an intensive program of education and role playing before they confront the alcoholic's problems directly. Its purpose is to prompt the alcoholic to accept treatment for chemical dependency by giving her or him a strong, well-coordinated push in that direction.

For most adolescents this form of structured intervention is too much, too soon. When interventions are done *incrementally*, starting with the least disruptive, time-consuming and expensive step, many young people are able to make necessary changes before more extreme steps must be taken.

For our purposes in this chapter, low-level interventions entail less time, money and disruption to a young person's life than high-level interventions. We try to show that even when a person does not benefit from a low-level intervention, behavior in that setting provides useful data for any future high-level intervention. In incremental intervention, then, assessment and intervention go hand-in-hand.

When intervention is assessment and vice versa

For some medical problems, diagnostic procedures and therapeutic procedures are one and the same. For instance, viral pneumonia may be indistinguishable from bacterial pneumonia until the patient fails to respond to antibiotics (in which case a virus is presumed to be the culprit). Similarly, estimation of the severity of a drug-use problem often proves difficult until the user attempts to stop using. Some young persons can make a contract with a counselor to refrain from using chemicals and their commitment to honesty will be sufficient to override their desire to take drugs. Others who make the same contract may be unable to abide by it, either because they are too heavily involved with drugs or because they are unable or unwilling to develop the kind of trust in relationships that makes such contracts meaningful. Who will abide by such a contract and who will not is a question that only time will answer.

Most professionals, no matter what their intuition tells them, want to give a young person some opportunity to work on staying drug free in a low-level intervention environment and avoid the considerable disruption that her or his removal from the community or prolonged absence from school would cause. Failure as well as success in such a setting contributes to the overall assessment process and provides specific behavioral data that help determine what types of additional help are needed.

The "hierarchy of interventions" outlined next is a method for reviewing each situation to determine what steps have been taken and what further steps must be taken to help a young person refrain from drug use.

A hierarchy of interventions

When discussing the range of possible interventions we could talk broadly about the various referral options available in the community: student support groups, outpatient family treatment, outpatient primary treatment for chemical dependency, inpatient treatment and long-term residential programs. The names of these basic services, however, do not describe the specific agents of change that contribute to the cessation of drug use and the alleviation of problems related to that use. The basic *agents of change* in a hierarchy of interventions are:

■ *Clarification of behavioral expectations.* Young people must be told by their parents, by school administrators and teachers, by counselors and by probation officers that drug use is not acceptable. This expectation has to be made explicit, and young people should know from experience that adults will back up what they say.

■ *Realistic information.* Young people must have a realistic understanding of the harmful effects of alcohol and other drugs.

■ *Personal awareness.* Young people should be made aware of the effects of their drug use on their own lives and the lives of family members and friends.

■ *Changes in the family system.* It may be necessary to intervene with a young person's family, altering those aspects of the system that contribute directly to his or her drug use or allow it to continue.

■ *Personal change.* Some young people need help for their psychological and emotional problems and difficulties with interpersonal relationships. Such help can range from a relatively low-level effort, such as classroom exercises on self-esteem, to high-level intervention, such as therapy focused on the person's fear of close relationships or distorted perceptions of reality. Personal change is always a major component of long-term (three- to six-month) residential treatment programs.

- **Direct, external control.** Some people need to have strict controls placed on them, perhaps entering a locked hospital ward or an inpatient treatment program far away from their own community, in order to be kept drug free long enough to develop the internal ability to refrain from drug use.

This list describes a "hierarchy" only in the most general sense. Broadly speaking, those interventions listed first are less intrusive and disruptive than those that follow. Each type of intervention can, of course, be implemented with varying degrees of intensity. Programs that imply a high level of intervention usually include several types of intervention. For instance, an inpatient chemical dependency treatment program that offers psychotherapy must also ensure that young clients understand the behavioral expectations of parents and schools. Treatment centers must also make certain that their young clients are not carrying around a great deal of misinformation about drugs.

This hierarchy of interventions implies a general sequence but does not mandate it. While it is best to see if a person will change when given appropriate information and when that person's awareness is increased, sometimes, almost paradoxically, the total process has to be reversed; a young person may first have to be physically removed from the drug-using environment and placed where drugs cannot be obtained. This person may also have to undergo intensive work on personality issues before she or he can benefit from information about drugs and their effect on his or her life. However, as we will see in the analysis of a school program in Chapter Nine, high-level interventions are needed much less often than low-level interventions.

None of the basic types of intervention have much chance of succeeding if a young person continues to use drugs while receiving assistance. While one of the most important goals of an early-intervention program is to help a young person develop the personal ability to refrain from drug use without constant external pressure and support, most programs usually apply external pressure and insist on abstinence during the first phases of intervention.

Clarification of behaviorial expectations

Many parents across the country are discovering that their children, even those as young as 12 or 13 years old, attend parties at which marijuana and alcohol are used. When they confront their children, parents are told this is the norm in their community and every party has some alcohol and marijuana use. Some parents have been successful at simply laying down the law and letting their children know that they may not go to such parties. Other parents have joined "parent peer groups" to decide what norms regarding parties they will enforce, where their children may congregate and what curfews will be imposed. The specification of clear behavioral norms has markedly limited drug abuse among certain peer groups and may even have prevented some young people from becoming dependent on chemicals.

Too many adults, it seems, fail to clarify behavioral expectations with young people because they do not feel it will do any good. Teachers who overhear references to a student being drunk at a party may fail to point out that drug and alcohol abuse is illegal, against school policies and likely to be very harmful to that person. Certainly, making young persons aware of these facts will not, in most cases, change their behavior. However, in some cases—1 of 10, 1 of 20 or 1 of 100—it may. Such a low-level intervention does not take much effort and may prompt a young person to think about whether or not to continue drug use. Furthermore, if all adults in a system—school, courts or social service—were to take the same stand, young people would begin to get the message that drug use by minors is not the norm and not acceptable to adults.

Some activities related to clarification of behavioral expectations are:

- *School policies and procedures*. When school policies and procedures are specific about what teachers and the rest of the staff will do when drug use is identified, students soon become aware of what behavior is expected. When school authorities apply these policies and procedures consistently, the policies and procedures stand a greater chance of being acted on by staff members and respected by students. The same applies to contracts between probation officers and their clients.

- *Parent/child communication*. Some structured methods can teach parents to be assertive and clear about their expectations of their children. The Parents Are Responsible (PAR) processes help accomplish this, as can other forms of communication training.

- *Parent peer groups*. As already mentioned, groups of parents can establish uniform community norms and commit themselves to enforcing them with their own children.

Realistic information about drug effects

Many professionals in the field believe that the abatement of the epidemic of amphetamine abuse in the early 1970s, the decline in the use of PCP in the mid-1970s and the decrease in marijuana use in the 1980s can all be attributed to the promulgation of realistic, honest information about the dangers of these drugs. We note that not only has overall marijuana use dropped but daily use has as well. The percentage of young people using marijuana daily has decreased by half, from 10.7% of all seniors in 1978 to 5.5% in 1983 (Johnston, O'Malley and Bachman, 1984).

Information, then, can be both a preventive agent and an intervention agent for drug problems. Even in intensive, inpatient treatment for heavy drug use, information about the effects of drugs on the body, mind and spirit are important contributors to the process of change. Whenever possible, we should try to provide drug abusers with the opportunity to change their behavior, based on a ra-

tional consideration of potential and actual effects of drugs on their lives.

Services that provide realistic information about drug effects include drug education in the classroom, literature on drugs and related problems, audiovisual materials and special events that help spread information about the effects of drugs. Sometimes information is offered to select groups of young people, for example, those who have violated drug use regulations.

Personal awareness of drug effects on one's own life

For a great many adults, this is *the* major agent of change. Once they really understand how their drug-related behavior has affected their loved ones, their jobs or their driving, they are ready to attempt to refrain from use of chemicals.

Schools and court services have a part to play in this type of intervention, but they can take it only so far. They can be very direct and insistent that young people be aware of data concerning school- and court-related behavior and can ask them to consider how drug use may be affecting their families and friends. However, some youth need intensive sessions with family members before they become truly aware of how they have affected their families. Such sessions are usually conducted outside of the school or court setting.

Here are some activities that stimulate the development of personal awareness of how drug use affects one's own life:

- *Insight Groups*. Described in Chapter Seven, Insight Groups are a means not only of providing information about drugs but of helping young people, through group processes and specific self-evaluation methods, to understand how drugs are affecting their lives.

- *General assessment procedures*. As data about a young person's problems accumulate during a general assessment, concerned adults and the young people themselves learn much about how drugs are affecting them and what other people think about it.

■ *Conferences*. Various conferences among parents, young people and other adults help to clarify the situation and confront young drug users with the need for change.

For young people who have developed the ability to maintain honest relationships with peers and adults and who have enough love and respect for themselves, the first three basic types of intervention have a strong possibility of succeeding. For people who do not respect themselves or others—because of a developmental lag or psychological problems or because drug use has superseded all other relationships—other interventions must be tried.

If the young person does not respond to clarification of behavioral expectations, to information about drug effects and to a personal examination of the effects of drugs on her or his own life, use of an in-depth assessment service, if available, may be necessary. Such an assessment agency uses both clinical techniques and information gained through the three intervention steps just described to determine what further action is warranted. The following intervention levels follow an intensive, thorough assessment process.

Changes in the family system

The young person should not be considered the sole source of the problem and the sole target of intervention if the family, school, community or any other overriding system is contributing to the problem. For example, if teachers have habitually ignored student drug use, it is hardly fair to suddenly start expelling students caught using or possessing alcohol or other drugs. The system that ignores, and thus allows, drug use must be altered before such heavy penalties are considered. So, too, the possibility of severe family disruption—physical abuse, incest, parental alcoholism and neglect—should be considered whenever heavy chemical dependency is encountered in adolescents. When inpatient treatment is necessary for such youths, treatment facilities with competence in family systems analysis and treatment should be

sought. Some services that can alter family systems are:

■ *Outpatient family treatment programs*. Whether drug-oriented or not, these programs employ a wide range of techniques to make families aware of and able to change the basic patterns of relationships that foster roles conducive to drug abuse.

■ *Outpatient and inpatient chemical dependency treatment programs*. Some treatment programs have a well-developed family component and deal with both problems simultaneously.

■ *Multiple-family therapy groups*. In these groups, one or two therapists work with five or six families together to alter family systems. This technique is employed in a variety of settings, including private practice by family therapists and structured treatment programs.

Personal Change

Sometimes young people need to build their self-esteem or improve their ability to form relationships before they can be expected to resist pressures to use drugs. This work often requires psychological and behavioral therapy.

When either the school system or the family system is dysfunctional, it is inappropriate to label the drug user as "the problem" and send him or her off to be treated individually. However, sometimes personal psychological problems occur in the absence of system dysfunction and must be taken care of. These problems can be a result of drug use, but most often they precede drug use. Resources relevant to intense personal change are:

■ *Long-term residential treatment programs*. These three- to six-month programs focus on basic behavioral change, self-awareness and personal responsibility. Group process, one-to-one counseling or therapy and the therapeutic milieu are all geared toward helping clients make basic changes in self-image and relationships with others.

■ *Long-term psychological or psychiatric treatment*.

Direct, external control

There are times when an adolescent must be removed from the school, from the home and even from the community to be given a "time-out" period in a drug-free environment before other interventions can begin. Those attempting to exert such control over adolescents should exert *legitimate power only*. If a student, whose life is not in immediate danger and who is not in danger of hurting another person, wishes to run out of the school while being confronted about drug use, school staff members probably have no right to restrain the student physically. We must all give up pretensions to power we do not have, while keeping all that is lawfully, ethically and professionally ours. (See "Intervention Means the Judicious Use of Legitimate Power" on page 56.)

Locked treatment wards, detoxification centers, juvenile centers and other forms of physical restraint are best used on a temporary basis only. Sometimes the very presence of a restraining option, such as a locked "quiet room" on an adolescent treatment unit, creates the need to use that room, either because clients unconsciously or consciously act in ways that force the staff to put them there or because the staff sees the need to resort to its use just because it exists. Nonetheless, external restraint of some kind is needed occasionally.

In sum, a mental checklist

The generic agents of change described by the hierarchy of interventions can serve as a simple checklist to keep in mind when we are faced with a drug-using adolescent. No matter what the setting—school, court, social service, inpatient treatment or home—we can review a series of questions that will point to the next step to be taken or retaken in an attempt to provide help. We can ask ourselves, "Does this person really know what behavior is expected by parents, the school and the courts? Does the person really believe that adults will do what they say they will do

if she or he uses drugs again? Does the person know what sniffing glue can do to the brain? Has the family system been investigated adequately to see if it could be a source of problems?"

Do not make presumptions! The question of whether or not a person has received the benefit from each type of intervention must be considered every time a young person is identified as having some sort of drug problem. We have already cited the very common problem of school drug policies that are never enforced. The mere existence of a policy tells us little or nothing about the actual message that students are getting about expected behavior. When policies are enforced and a person has been offered a service, we cannot presume that she or he has derived the maximum potential benefit from that service. If, for example, a young man was involved in a support group to help him become aware of how drugs were affecting his life but was too angry or immature at the time to derive any benefit, he probably did not give himself an opportunity to learn how drugs were actually affecting him and his relationships. If he has matured since the time of the original group, it may be that he could benefit from another try at such an intervention rather than moving immediately to a more intrusive and disruptive intervention. A regular review of the incremental components of the early-intervention process can be formalized in program evaluations or research projects. Its more practical application, however, would be to serve as a simple guideline, a mental checklist, to help in daily work with troubled young people.

It is best for front-line people, such as teachers and coaches who work with a fairly large number of young people every day, to avoid becoming too wrapped up in trying to determine what types of intervention have been tried with a young person. The job of front-line people is identification and initial action. Determination of the next appropriate step to take is the responsibility of an early-intervention counselor. Indecision on the part of the identifiers should not cause a delay in obtaining help for troubled youths.

Intervention by Juvenile Justice and Social Service Systems

Everyone has a role to play in helping young people and adults refrain from harmful drug use. Since this book is oriented toward program planning, we focus on system-wide approaches rather than personal, one-to-one approaches. We directly address three basic systems: the juvenile justice systems, the social service agencies and the schools. Each system has various advantages and disadvantages for early intervention, depending on a wide variety of factors, including:

o the portion of the population of young people with which the system works;

o the level of intervention called for by the young person's history and present situation;

o motivational factors of the young person and the leverage available to the particular system in question; and

o early-intervention capability: the specific early-intervention services—identification, initial response, preliminary assessment, etc.—that the system can offer.

Let us first look at juvenile justice and social service systems and see the strengths and weaknesses each has for implementing early-intervention services.

Juvenile justice systems

Special population
Juvenile courts serve a unique population of young people. First, the courts are likely to reach some young people who are not even present in other systems. Some school dropouts, for instance, who are not reachable through school-based early-intervention programs will be involved with the legal system. Second, the rate of drug-use problems among court-referred populations appears to be much greater than among the general popu-

lation of young people. As one probation officer put it, "It's my feeling that just about every kid we see in court is involved with chemicals to some extent. Almost every kid arrested has either experimented with drugs, has a problem with them or comes from a home with a drug problem."

The state of Wisconsin studied 1,185 juveniles who were held in temporary "secure detention" for up to 24 hours (Halikas, Lyttle, Morse and Hoffmann, 1984). These were juveniles who had not yet been convicted of a current crime but were being held for "probable cause." This meant that they were suspected of having committed an act of delinquency or a status offense and either had a past history of failure to adhere to juvenile court actions, were fugitives or were identified as repeated runaways. This group of juvenile detainees did not report drinking at a higher rate than that of the general youth population, but did report more consequences relative to drinking. Of the 1,185 subjects interviewed, 82% reported having used alcohol and 71% of the drinkers reported negative consequences. The following is a description of the general problem areas considered in the study; figures in parentheses indicate the proportion of drinkers in the study manifesting symptoms in each problem area:

■ *Psychosocial complications (55%)*. This could include a family member expressing concern; drinking at home in front of parents; no non-drinking friends; drinking patterns causing family fights or arguments; problems with parents or friends because of alcohol; treatment for alcohol abuse; and arrests related to alcohol.

■ *Biomedical complications (52%)*. This could include behavior changes due to alcohol use; memory blackouts due to alcohol; morning drinking; hallucinations due to alcohol; and shakes due to alcohol.

■ *School problems (34%)*. This could include drinking while truant; drinking on school grounds; school absences due to intoxication

Intervention Means the Judicious Use of Legitimate Power

In assessment and intervention, we have to know what power people have and what power they are willing to use. Some sources of power are:

○ *Personal power voluntarily given by young drug users to others*. A younger sister may have power because an older sibling who is using drugs does not want to hurt her anymore or parents may have power because a drug-using son or daughter still loves them.

○ *Community standards*. It is an accepted norm in most communities that until a young person leaves home parents have the right to limit his or her behavior in various ways.

○ *State and federal laws*. School officials, parents and other adults are lawfully charged with certain responsibilities for minors as well as some authority to carry out those responsibilities.

○ *Forfeited power*. Some youths have lost certain privileges and thus have forfeited their power of self-determination. An adolescent who has smashed up a car while drunk has clearly given up not only the right to drive a car but, if there were serious injuries, other personal freedoms as well. She or he may be incarcerated for a time and treatment for drug problems can be made a requirement of probation or parole.

It is best to base interventions on the power freely granted by the drug abuser rather than on power that is more coercive in nature. When counselors try to use power not legitimately theirs, such as not letting a young person out of a locked room until he or she has listened to all the data, they may violate ethical, professional and/or legal codes. Again, the power used in interventions should be legitimate power only.

or hangover; drinking in school buildings; keeping alcohol in the school; needing a drink before going to school; or being seen by a social worker or counselor because of drinking.

In order to receive a diagnosis of "alcohol abuser," a subject had to have at least one symptom in each of the three problem areas. Even using these stringent criteria for diagnosis, 19% of all subjects and 24% of the drinkers were diagnosed as alcohol abusers. The average number of symptoms manifested by those receiving a positive diagnosis was seven. Bear in mind that this pertains only to alcohol use. Although the findings relevant to the use of other drugs were not included in the published article, our personal correspondence with the agency at which the study took place indicates that at least 30% of the court population would receive a diagnosis of either alcohol or drug abuser if drugs other than alcohol were figured into the equation.

Compared with short-term juvenile detainees, those in long-term detention might well be expected to exhibit a higher incidence of drug and alcohol problems. This suspicion is corroborated by a study of the state training school in Red Wing, Minnesota (Sipe and Hunter, 1980), in which a chemical use survey was administered to 100 residents. The survey emphasized chemical use history, family intactness and support systems, self-concepts and self-esteem, negative consequences related to use and programming needs. Staff members were also interviewed concerning their perceptions of the problem and were asked about the need for specialized programs. In addition, 30% of the case files were randomly selected and scrutinized for consequences of chemical use. Overall, Sipe and Hunter found that:

○ 75% of the residents surveyed reported that they had experienced negative consequences as a result of their use of chemicals.
○ 57% reported daily use of marijuana. This is more than *six times* the incidence of daily marijuana use (9.1%) reported by the general

student population of the United States in that same year, 1980 (Johnston, Bachman and O'Malley, 1982b).

○ 53% of the residents reported that they had been using or were high on chemicals at the time they were arrested for the crime that resulted in their current incarceration.
○ 40% of the juveniles released from the institution are paroled to chemical dependency programs.
○ 39% of the residents surveyed had seen a counselor because of their chemical use or had been in chemical dependency treatment. This is *eight times* the incidence reported by the general student population of Minnesota (Benson, et al., 1983).
○ 21% reported daily use of alcohol. This is more than *three times* the incidence of daily use (6%) reported by the general student population of the United States in 1980 (Johnston et al., 1982b).

Stage of intervention

Since court services tend to identify youths who are heavily involved with drugs, a higher level of intervention is usually called for. For instance, the proportion of referrals from court services who go to inpatient treatment is greater than that of referrals from schools. (See Chapter Ten for a review of referral patterns from the courts.)

Motivation and leverage

The courts have a great deal of leverage in obtaining cooperation from young people and their families. Many therapists have had clients who simply did not work at all in treatment until they got a clear message from a probation officer, who said that if they did not cooperate their next stop would be juvenile detention.

Extreme caution must be used here, however. The juvenile detention system, especially the long-term institutionalization of young offenders, has been very destructive for many young people. If the local legal system is not adequate (as in those cases where juveniles are incarcerated with adults), use of court services in drug-related situations is probably too dangerous. If, however, court services are clearly humane and many safeguards are in place, the leverage provided by firm but fair court action can motivate young people to participate in other intervention services.

Early-intervention capabilities

In terms of the six basic processes of early intervention, juvenile justice services are very well equipped to offer identification, initial action and some preliminary assessment services. Identification services are crucial because the incidence of drug use among court clients is so high. Initial action by court personnel can have a strong impact on young people, who are usually quite willing to cooperate with court staff. In the process of pretrial screenings and presentence investigations, the courts have leverage to direct other family members, school authorities and mental health centers to provide information useful for preliminary assessments. Information gathered in court investigations is sometimes sufficient in and of itself or can contribute to assessments carried out by the schools or other agencies.

Regarding support for change, probation officers can play an important role, although preferably not by themselves, in supporting those of their clients who have decided to commit themselves to drug-free living.

Social service agencies

Special population

Social service agencies, such as welfare and child protection units, sometimes treat unique populations, each of which may exhibit a higher incidence of drug use than the general population. As is true of the courts, social service agencies can identify and assist young people who have dropped out of school and therefore cannot be reached by school-based programs.

Social service agencies also serve many troubled adults. Since these adults are often parents, it is likely that the children of those in need of social services are at greater risk of drug use. This, of course, depends on the nature of the agency.

Stage of intervention

While courts usually intervene with young people whose level of drug use is relatively high and schools intervene with a range of users, it is harder to make such general statements about social service agencies as a group. Child abuse services, for instance, may encounter more drug problems among victims and their siblings than general welfare services do.

Motivation and leverage

Various social service agencies may or may not have the direct leverage that the courts and, in some cases, the schools have. When the courts apply pressure, however, the agencies are given additional leverage for working with less motivated, less cooperative clients.

Although leverage might be absent, some clients will want to work with a social service agency if they are convinced that some of their problems will be addressed.

Early-intervention capabilities

Welfare and child protection services are in particularly good positions for identifying and offering initial aid to young drug users and young people being adversely affected by the chemical use of a family member. The types of situational and long-term problems presented to such agencies are often, though certainly not always, related to the drug and alcohol problems of parents. The data gathered by staff members who work with family problems can also be helpful in a preliminary or in-depth assessment process conducted by a school or drug assessment service. Because of budgetary restraints and severe time pressure put on staff members, most welfare and child protection agencies may find it difficult to develop their own formal assessment programs.

Social service agencies may also be able to offer some support for clients who attempt to refrain from drug use.

Community mental health centers can also play varying roles in all six early-intervention processes—identification, initial action, preliminary assessment, referral, some direct service in the broad continuum of care and support for change. A crucial point to keep in mind is that no matter how good the quality of their services, the scope of the services these multifaceted agencies can offer is limited and those limits should be recognized. In regard to identification of drug problems, they identify only those problems present among their clients and do not reach a broad spectrum of youth in the community. Furthermore, in offering direct services to people, these agencies must not try to be the only service provider for all the problems that are uncovered; they should expect to refer clients to other agencies when they themselves cannot offer the best service for a given problem.

***   ***   ***

Incremental intervention and ongoing assessment are the heart and soul of early intervention. Juvenile justice and social service agencies can contribute to the incremental intervention process at various times in a young person's life. In the next chapter, we show that schools are extremely well situated to contribute to this process at virtually every stage in a young person's life, from the first time a student is likely to feel pressure to try alcohol and other drugs to the threshold of adulthood.

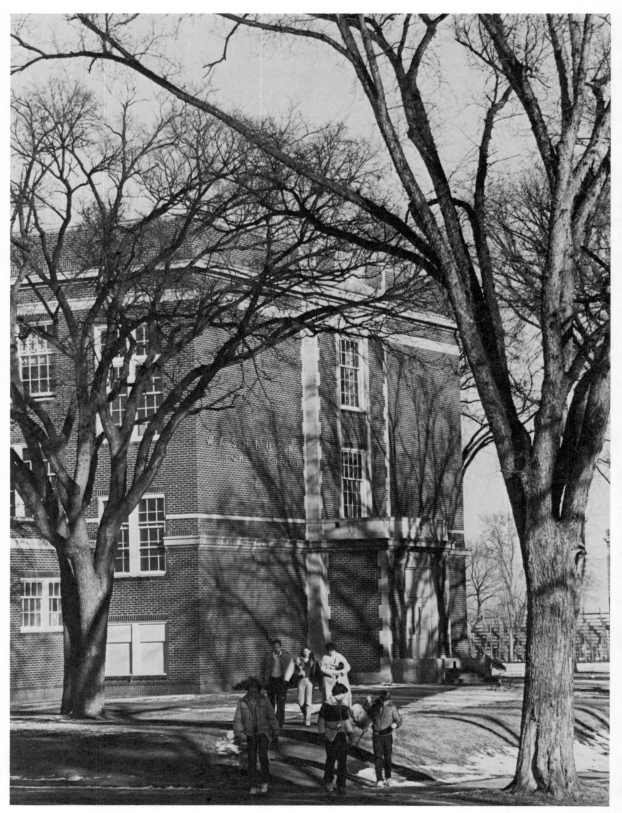

photo: Joseph Muldoon

CHAPTER FIVE

REACHING THOSE IN NEED
The School's Advantages

At 7:45 on a Friday morning, John Frederickson, math teacher at Miskatonic High School, parks his car in the faculty parking lot and walks toward the infamous north door. It faces Fairview Avenue, where, it is generally known, the "druggies" hang out before class. Although a few students have been arrested or otherwise disciplined for drinking alcohol or smoking marijuana there, the administration and teachers have been reluctant to apply more pressure lest they uncover problems they are not ready to handle, such as having to call in the police, or having to answer to the public as to why nothing was done before.

As Mr. Frederickson ascends the stairway into the building, he notices one of his better students talking with a group of kids strongly suspected of using drugs. In a split second, he assesses the situation and makes his choice. An expanded version of his internal monologue might run something like this:

"Hey, that's Tommy Johnson and I think he has a joint. Now if I stop and ask him if he's holding some drug, he'll say no. I can't make him show it to me and I don't think we're allowed to search students. Anyway, he was out on Fairview Avenue, wasn't he? Doesn't that mean the school isn't involved?

"Anyway, Tommy's a pretty good kid and you never know how the assistant principal is going to handle it. The least he'll do is kick him out for ten days, and if the administration thinks that drug use is getting out of hand again, he might recommend expulsion just to make an example of him.

"Besides, no one has hassled the kids at the north door for a long time. This is no man's land. I'd be the only one on the staff sticking my neck out. I know Tommy wouldn't do anything, but those other guys would. I might find my tires flat when I leave tonight.

"I think, maybe, when I get a chance, I'll talk to Tommy confidentially. Won't see him today, though.

"This'll teach me to come through that damned north door in the morning. Tomorrow I'm going to get here five minutes earlier so I have time to go around to the front door."

The sort of split-second decision that John Frederickson made is not uncommon. He is *not* in favor of alcohol or marijuana use by teenagers. He thinks the drugs *are* harmful to students, but he still does not act. If we look at what went through his mind during the split second in which he made his decision, we see that (1) he was not sure of the school policy on drug use near the school and did not know the procedure to follow concerning possession of drugs by a student; (2) he was not sure that the administration would be fair and consistent in dealing with Tommy; (3) he did not believe in the policy of a ten-day suspension with no other services being offered; (4) he reacted to the general unsafe, untrusting climate in the school, believing his car would be vandalized if he tried to act against the drug problem; (5) he thought that he had an alternative that would do just as much good, that of talking to Tommy confidentially about his problem.

Obviously, whether or not Miskatonic High School has a policy and/or a program relevant to drug problems, Mr. Frederickson is profoundly affected by the problem. If there is a policy, Mr. Frederickson clearly was not involved in its formulation and whoever formulated it has not assured its implementation in any useful fashion.

Schools offer exceptional opportunities for early intervention into drug problems. As the preceding example demonstrates, however, people do not always make good use of these opportunities. There were various courses of action that the beleaguered math teacher could have taken, and there is no single answer to the problem he faced. In Chapter Six we describe some of those options in the section "Initial Action." The reason that he decided to take no action at all, however, was because he felt isolated. He did not know of any clear, comprehensive approach agreed to by his peers and supervisors. He knew bits and pieces of the school policy, but they did not make sense to him. In Miskatonic High School, then, there was little shared understanding of the basics of drug problems and no consensus as to what early-intervention techniques were to be employed.

In this chapter we present some material that can help in building a consensus about a general, school-based approach to drug problems. We consider the necessity of schools becoming involved in early-intervention programs; the various advantages and drawbacks; and the typical evolution in schools from no programs to effective broad-based early-intervention strategies.

The School's Investment in Early Intervention

To understand why schools should be interested in early-intervention programming, we have to look beyond ideology and philosophy and consider the practical realities of drug use in the school setting.

Avoid rigid philosophical stands

Making absolute definitions of the school's role in working with adolescent drug and alcohol abuse problems is not difficult. Making these definitions work in the real world is difficult. Some people base their arguments on abstract ideals. Schools, they say, exist solely to teach; schools can, therefore, disseminate information about drugs and provide growth experiences that reinforce prevention, but preliminary assessment and intervention are not part of the school's role. Other agencies, they say, can do that job.

Such philosophical stands on the ideal role of schools must inevitably be balanced against practical and pragmatic considerations. These vary from one school district to the next. Sparsely populated areas, for example, do not usually have a range of agencies competent to deal with drug problems. If, by chance or by training, schools happen to have personnel with the talent, insight and skills to assist young people, should they refuse to do so on the basis of general ideals? If schools wait for floundering agencies to develop skills, many students with problems will not get the help they need. And then, when other agencies do develop services, they often cannot reach students in the early stages of their problems.

In many communities, schools are the only central locations linked by convenient transportation services. Insight Groups could be sponsored by many community agencies, but how would students get there and back? Would students have to arrange for their own transportation? Would this inconvenience or discourage many of them? Such simple, practical factors as transportation often tip the balance in favor of schools being the ideal sites for many early-intervention activities.

Direct effects of drug problems

In Chapter Three we cited a study sponsored by the federal government (Rachal et al., 1982) in which students who had become harmfully involved with drugs (31.2% of the students in the sample) admitted to having, much more frequently than other students, "trouble with teachers or principals, difficulties with friends, driving after having a 'good bit' to drink, criticism from a date and trouble with the police." All these trouble areas could involve difficulty at school or school-sponsored events.

Another trouble area is academic performance. Cooper, Olson and Fournier (1977) reported "a significant relationship between drug use and grades." Those students in this study identified as "frequent users" (using at least one drug four or more times per week) were the only group who received a sizeable proportion of Ds or Fs. The general findings of poor academic performance among frequent drug users upheld those of a 1976 study by Anhalt and Klein. It does not matter whether poor grades are a cause or an effect of drug use. The simple likelihood of a relationship between drug use and grades should be of concern to school personnel.

An article by Cohen and Santo (1977) contained the following highlights, which should be of interest to educators:

○ In a study of students in Boise, Idaho, only 3.75% of the students with an A grade average were current users of marijuana, whereas 100% of those with a D average reported current marijuana use.

○ Another study showed that of 2,750 young people aged 12 to 19 who had been admitted to some type of drug abuse program, 715 (26%) were school dropouts. Since this study included kids of junior high school age, it is likely that by the time they reached age 18 or older, the dropout rate would have been con-

siderably higher. The study also found that 64% of those in treatment who were age 17 or older were behind the grade level appropriate for their age.

○ Among 8,553 students in New York State public schools, the incidence of abstinence from chemicals was three times higher for students with "high interest" in school than for students with "low interest." Furthermore, 9.1% of "low interest" students had tried five to seven mood-altering substances in their lives, compared with only 1.9% of the "high interest" students.

Keep in mind that these findings are only the hard data. Anecdotal information from hundreds of teachers and other school staff members has convinced us that the use of alcohol and other drugs is having a powerful effect on the educational process in this country. Your own efforts to obtain anecdotal information will probably reap the same response. Guidelines for gathering useful anecdotal data, which is an important part of a needs assessment for community and school programming, are described in *Alliance for Change* by James Crowley.

Special opportunities to help

There is a difference between the *schools' responsibilities* and the *schools' opportunities*. For example, some people may question whether or not it is the schools' responsibility to identify children of alcoholics who are not progressing adequately in school. Schools do, however, have a rare opportunity, unmatched by that of any other agency or institution in the community, to be helpful in this area (see Chapter Seven). To let such an opportunity pass could well mean that many children will leave the school system and grow to adulthood without ever being given help for what is probably the single most important issue in their lives. The young people who are suffering, their families and their future families would miss a tremendous opportunity.

Let us look at the goals of early-intervention programs and consider the advantages that schools offer for helping young people with problems:

- *Identification of troubled students*. Schools work with virtually *every* child in the community at one time or another. Thus, they are the ideal institutions to help identify young people with drug use and related problems.

- *Initial action*. Schools are in a unique position to motivate students and parents to take action on their own or to cooperate with actions initiated by others. Most students are motivated to stay in school, whether because of academic aspirations, the need to socialize or the desire to participate in extracurricular activities. When remaining in school is contingent on their cooperation with early-intervention activities, grudging cooperation is usually forthcoming. Even when students are not under any outside pressure to cooperate with the school, the fact that program staff members are readily accessible, at least for brief periods during the day, makes it easier for young people to take the first, frightening step of asking for help. In well-developed programs, where trust is high and students and staff members are familiar with program services, it is not uncommon for students to pressure their peers into participating in the program when they think it can do some good.

- *Preliminary assessment and data gathering*. The structured setting of schools provides a unique opportunity for preliminary screening and assessment. The clear criteria of compulsory attendance and academic performance provide generally accepted reference points for evaluation of recent changes and current functioning. Even parents do not have these criteria available to them at home because they often do not know what life is like in other families. Unlike schools, community agencies tend to deal only with those young people whose problems have become so severe as to overcome the normal reluctance of parents to seek help from professionals.

- *Referral options*. Schools have a unique advantage when it comes to the type and timing of referrals made for young drug users. Since schools are appropriate and convenient locations for a variety of awareness, education and abstinence support groups, these services can be used as first-time, low-level interventions to make young people aware of their reasons for using drugs and of the effects that drug use is having in their lives. Furthermore, since the school staff members see students daily, they are in an excellent position to monitor behavior when a question of drug use arises. This helps avoid the necessity of having to decide immediately about referral when a person's situation is unclear and more data are needed. Fuzzy cases can be watched closely until data accumulate and clarify the need or lack of need for outside assistance.

- *Continuum of care*. Many of the services that are necessary for dealing with young drug users cannot and should not be offered by schools. Nonetheless, schools can take an active role in the development of community services. As we have mentioned previously, schools that have been able to describe the unmet needs of students have been a major force in getting those services developed in their communities.

- *Support for change*. Since peer pressure to use drugs is strong in school and at school-related activities, support services provided right at this "pressure point" can help students maintain the changes they have made in treatment, in self-help programs or in counseling.

When schools take on tasks that have more to do with opportunities than responsibilities, the community should take note and offer support. Certainly, the educational process will benefit as drug problems are alleviated, and it is thus appropriate that a certain amount of school funds be allocated to this task. However, support from the community—volunteer time, contributions from businesses, state aid and foundation grants—is consistent with the notion that this is a community-wide project and that schools are definitely helping the community by serving as the focal point for early intervention.

Typical Program Evolution

School-based early-intervention programs typically start with a strong emphasis on students who actually use drugs on the premises but those programs move quickly into other areas. As the problem focus expands, so do the methods of identification and initial action.

Stages in evolution

Once established, most drug programs undergo a natural process of evolution. To quote from one evaluation study (Larsen, 1982), "As the chemical dependency counselors gained experience in working with this student group, it became apparent that there existed a cluster of related problems that must be dealt with; these include abuse, neglect, family relationships and incest. The current program has evolved to address not only chemical issues but these related concerns as well."

In the first stage of development, then, programs are primarily reactive, trying to play catch-up when school personnel identify more problems than the staff of the early-intervention program can handle. In later stages, after early-intervention programs have been in place for several years, they move toward the pro-active student assistance model.

The "reactive" or "catch-up" program

In the first stage, many programs find themselves reacting primarily to cases generated by disciplinary procedures. The general objective of such a program may read: "To assess and refer for help those students who violate school regulations or state, local and federal laws related to the possession or selling of drugs on school grounds or at school events."

This is not a very comprehensive goal. Nonetheless, it is a legitimate goal and often takes up a great deal of time in any program in the early stage of development. This kind of program is often the result of an abrupt decision in the school or community to "get tough on drug abuse." If school authorities have decided to suspend many more students for use, possession or selling on school grounds, it behooves some staff members to be around to deal with the fallout from this decision.

There are some serious drawbacks to this reactive approach, especially if the consequences of getting caught are extremely harsh, indiscriminate and punitive. A student who has been suspended for a month or expelled until the end of the year for alcohol or drug use is unlikely to be very cooperative with the assessment and referral process. The purpose of a preliminary assessment is not only to get some idea of the nature and extent of a young person's problems but also to make the person aware of the potential for problems in the future, of the general need for immediate action and of the specific type of action needed now. The assessment serves to demonstrate both to parents and to their children just how drug use is hurting them and what has to be done. Part of the assessment process, then, is educating people about the nature of their problems and some options for solving them. If the early-intervention program becomes too closely associated with disciplinary mechanisms in the school, the program may acquire a stigma that works against cooperation, and people may defiantly refuse to take advantage of the services available to them.

When a program is playing catch-up, the early-intervention process is not so much active as it is reactive. It is not seeking out the students who most need help but instead is dealing with those who rise to the surface because of their flamboyant behavior. Catch-up programs are likely to deal with more boys than girls. In terms of the general program objectives, identification is left to outside forces and assessment takes on a different tone than it otherwise would.

Common Program Components

The goals of early intervention determine the types of staff members needed to work in the program and the types of activities undertaken. The following activities are common to most school-based early-intervention programs:

o *Policies and procedures* on how to deal with student chemical use, behavior that is being affected by drug use and other associated personal problems are drawn up, publicized and consistently followed.

o *A core team* made up of school staff members should plan and develop the program and carry out many of the activities. Administrators, noncertified staff members, teachers, coaches, nurses and counselors should all be represented on the team. Very small districts have one core team for the entire district, but others have a core team for each building or building complex. In many schools, core team members are the only people who have access to confidential information gained during the intervention process.

o *A program coordinator* should be designated. In smaller programs, this job is usually handled by a counselor or teacher who squeezes coordinator duties into an already packed schedule. As programs grow, a half- to full-time coordinator is usually needed.

o *An advisory board* should be made up of a wide range of people from the school district and the community. Parents, school board members, business people, students and professional service providers are usually represented.

o *Training* for core team and advisory board members is crucial to engender enthusiasm among those working in or supporting the program and to develop specific skills in program management, preliminary assessment, community education and other activities.

o *An assessment system* provides efficient, consistent, high-quality preliminary assessment services to students (see Chapter Seven).

o *A variety of support groups* can be offered to help students who have problems with drug use, students who are trying to maintain drug-free lifestyles and students who are being affected by the drug use of others. In addition to these basic groups, schools may offer other services when the need arises (see Chapter Seven).

o *A budget* should clearly allot funds for personnel, staff training and other activities or materials. Integration with the school's budget makes the early-intervention program part of the organizational structure and thus more likely to last.

Drug assessment as an adjunct to a more comprehensive process

Some early-intervention programs focus exclusively on alcohol and drug use, leaving the identification and assessment of other problems to preexisting systems in the school. Some schools, for example, rely on child-study teams consisting of a social worker, psychologist, counselor and special education teacher to screen students for other problems that may be affecting their personal, social and educational development. In these schools, a drug-oriented early-intervention program is an adjunct to a more comprehensive assessment process.

Early-intervention staff members should never assume that preexisting mechanisms are reliable. It is better to test to see whether problems are actually being uncovered by other school services. Simple screening questions for family problems, such as abuse and incest, should be asked of all students entering the drug program, at least for a time.

Drug awareness/student assistance as a pro-active approach

Pro-active programs start by taking a positive approach to identification and initial action. They try to reach those young people most in need, even if some are not likely to come forward on their own or be referred by an adult. This means being sensitive and responsive to all kinds of behavior indicative of personal, family and drug problems.

In pro-active programs, patterns of identification and initial action are closely monitored, as are the assessment process and referrals to community resources. The program evaluation formats have specific goals based on the estimated number of young people who are using drugs and who are in trouble with drugs; the programs seek to discern not only those who are already being referred but also those who are *not* being referred. Based on other observations and program records, staff members look at whether minorities are coming through; whether a disproportionate number of boys or girls are coming through;

and whether these patterns relate to actual patterns of drug use or to quirks in the program. Staff members also attempt to identify actual problems and potential problems earlier and are more active in soliciting information from teachers as cases emerge.

Student assistance programs: the natural development

When the concept of employee assistance programs first took hold among employers, there was a vehement outcry from the people in charge of alcohol programs in business and industry. They feared, among other things, that programs established to deal with a wide range of problems would neglect alcoholics. They also feared that alcoholism professionals would lose their positions to mental health professionals. Both fears proved unfounded. Occupational program consultants found that when employee assistance programs employed professionals competent in the area of drug and alcohol abuse, alcoholics were not ignored and continued to be identified and helped as before. In fact, since the employee assistance programs were open to a wide range of presenting complaints, including marital, financial and legal problems, some industrial counselors felt they were identifying problem drinkers earlier because these other problems were often related to drinking.

Experience with school-based early-intervention programs indicates that this same pattern is being played out again. It appears that in programs that have been in existence for a number of years, "student assistance programs" and "chemical awareness programs" tend to work with similar proportions of drug abusers, children from alcoholic families and students with other problems. You cannot tell a book by its cover or a program by its label. A student assistance program may devote all efforts to drug-related issues, while many chemical awareness programs work well with a wide range of problems.

When alcohol and drug programs evolve

into broad-based student assistance programs, they must be ready and willing to deal with any problems that come their way, including physical abuse, incest and concerns about sexual identity. Most programs, however, will continue to place considerable emphasis on identifying and assisting students with chemical-related problems. Some readers may wonder, "Why should this emphasis be maintained? Why don't schools have special incest programs or physical abuse programs, for example?"

These are good questions and the point is well taken, but whether we call a program a chemical dependency program, a chemical awareness program or student assistance program, the following compelling reasons to develop strong competencies in matters related to drug abuse remain:

▪ *There is a great amount of school-related drug activity*. Schools are the place to buy, the place to sell and the place to use drugs. Young people do not gather at the psychology clinic or the juvenile court to hang around and find drugs. Because schools are an incubation point for many drug problems, they are an appropriate place for prevention and intervention efforts.

▪ *Drug problems spread in the school environment*. Problems such as incest and child abuse do not spread through peer pressure in the school environment. Drug problems do.

▪ *Drugs can be the preferred "calling card" for other personal problems*. As we have noted, an abused teenager is quite likely to use chemicals. It may be easier for that student to admit to drug use to a counselor than to disclose other problems that may be considered more shameful. In fact, some counselors have observed that when drug use is the problem, the person hides it, and when other problems are more important, drug use is flaunted.

▪ *Drug problems can be symptomatic of other serious problems*. This fact is actually a good reason for making drug problems the program's focus. Schools with clear criteria for

dealing with adolescent drug problems are likely to identify more abused children and children with emotional problems than schools without drug programs that try, in a variety of other ways, to help the abused and emotionally neglected.

▪ *Adolescent drug problems provide the best rallying point for establishing both student assistance and chemical awareness programs*. The problem of adolescent drug abuse has seized the nation's interest, especially the interest of parents groups. This is a notable phenomenon. It means that while many communities may still avoid the issue of child abuse and other problems of dysfunctional families, they are likely to be willing to confront drug problems. Every community mobilization project needs a "handle," a visible rallying point for action. Drug abuse provides the strongest and clearest motivation for establishing early-intervention programs that can deal with a range of problems.

In summary, then, drug problems can be the primary focus of early-intervention programs without excluding other problems. Once the mechanisms for early intervention have been established, a variety of student problems can be identified and referred for assistance with little increase in the amount of time and money needed.

Some limitations

Although schools have many advantages in identifying and screening young people who have drug problems, they also have some intrinsic limitations.

Schools are definitely not in the treatment business and school staff members should not attempt to act as therapists. Clear-cut policies and procedures related to drug use can keep teachers from taking on the role of drug counselor. As mentioned before, in a well-implemented early-intervention program, teachers and other front-line staff members are asked to refrain both from attempting to diagnose problems and from doing too much counseling. Serious drug problems are to be moved out of the school into an appropriate assessment, counseling or treatment setting without delay. Less serious problems may be dealt with in-house in a consistent and efficient manner using school-based services delivered by trained staff members.

In practical terms, outside agencies are becoming more important to school programs as funding cuts begin to hit schools harder. Whether support groups are held in the school or in a local agency, it has become more common for group leadership to be shared by a school employee and a professional from an outside agency.

Also, issues of confidentiality become more complex in the school setting, where a variety of state and federal laws may apply. Sometimes, but not always, an agency outside the school has more freedom to share information among family members than school staff members operating under school policies do.

Despite these limitations, school early-intervention personnel must still learn about the full range of assessment and referral techniques, even if much of this work is to be done by an outside agency. If schools intend to make referrals to outside agencies, they have a responsibility to make certain that those agencies are at least meeting the minimum requirements of competent service.

* * *   * * *   * * *

The schools do have an investment in early intervention as well as definite strengths for implementing such programs. In the next chapter we see, in practical terms, how schools, courts and social service agencies can capitalize on their strengths.

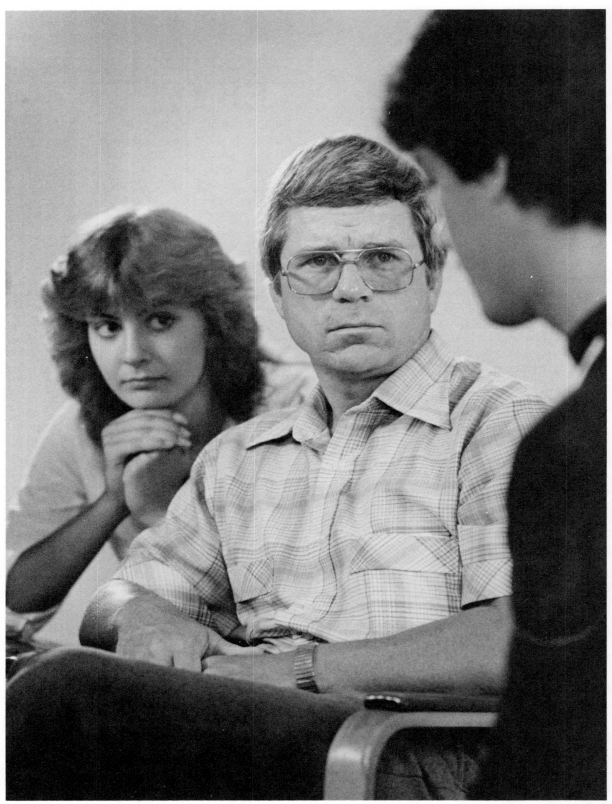

photo: Jeffrey Grosscup

CHAPTER SIX

EFFECTIVE INTERVENTION
The First Three Steps

It is not uncommon for counselors to feel insecure when asked to make decisions about young drug users. This insecurity usually arises not so much from a lack of clinical skills or knowledge about young people and drugs as from the kinds of questions asked and the nature of the decisions required before sufficient information becomes available. For instance, when a student is suspected of being "high" at school, the principal may ask, "Is this kid chemically dependent?" Often, this question is asked because there are services for chemical dependency but not for other types of problems related to drug use. For a great many reasons, however, this question is frequently impossible to answer within a short period. Any conscientious counselor would find the task very difficult. What may feel to the counselor like a lack of interviewing skills is really a function of the haphazard method by which young people are referred, the fuzzy data that accompany referrals, the limited options for action and problems caused by the over-application of the concept of adolescent chemical dependency.

There is no magic in the assessment of drug problems. Most schools, court services and social service providers have staff members who are competent in interviewing and counseling young people and their families.

If the referral system is well organized, these people can do preliminary assessments of and make decisions about young people. The effectiveness of preliminary assessments depends on what types of problems are identified, what steps are taken before a person is interviewed and how data are gathered from various sources.

This chapter focuses on practical techniques for identifying drug problems, taking initial action and gathering information. These three steps of early intervention are almost entirely dependent on front-line people who work with young people every day, whereas assessment of referral data, interviewing and facilitation of support groups are the responsibilities of specially-trained core team members of the programs. (Interviewing and support groups are discussed in Chapter Seven.) How well core team members and special program counselors are able to train and communicate with school or agency staff members as a whole determines the effectiveness of identification, initial action and data-gathering procedures.

Many of the general factors contributing to the early-intervention process are summarized in Chapter Eleven, "Program Review: Back to the Basics." A clear, mutual understanding of the basic premises concerning adolescent drug use and early intervention, pre-

Adolescent Drug Users' Techniques to Avoid Being Identified

Some young people use drugs to mask personal pain. Often, these are the kids who do something quite obvious to get caught so that they can obtain help for problems other than drug use. Unlike these kids are those youths who are highly invested in protecting their drug use. Some of their techniques to avoid detection, as revealed to a school counselor in a survey of kids in an aftercare group, are:

○ *Be ingratiating.* Some have found it very effective to get on the good side of teachers and butter them up.

○ *Never use in school, but use heavily elsewhere.* Some young people have enough control to play this game well.

○ *Stay stoned.* Some kids are high so much of the time that adults believe the symptoms are just part of their lethargic or detached nature.

○ *Act dumb.* When students cannot keep up with activities because they are stoned, they simply act as though the material is too hard for them and elicit help from teachers.

○ *Lie low.* A good ploy is to never ask questions, never act out, never come to the attention of adults in any way.

○ *Have plenty of reasonable explanations.* Excuses for drug-induced symptoms can range from being tired from work, to being mildly sick, to having difficulty with contact lenses.

○ *Be a fast talker.* Some kids are really good at thinking on their feet. If teachers, coaches, administrators or probation officers ask them to explain their behavior, they can come up with a variety of explanations that cover all bases.

○ *Find a weakness in the system.* Many students go to the nurse's office to avoid classes and to sleep off the effects of drugs.

○ *Take advantage of department isolation.* Teachers from different departments may not talk to one another or check up when students give them excuses. Students become aware of just how this lack of communication works and are willing to use it.

○ *Forge passes.*

○ *Be compliant.* Doing whatever a teacher says, or at least acting agreeable, wards off confrontation.

○ *Lie and tell half-truths.* Outright deception continues to work well.

○ *Write your own excuses.* Older students often get away with writing their own excuses for absences or for passes.

sented there and in previous chapters, should result in the development of better and more consistent assessment procedures.

Identification

In this section we review the major target groups for early intervention and consider some methods that have been used to facilitate the identification of young people in need of services.

Target groups

No matter where a program stands in its evolution from reactive to pro-active, program staff members should try to conceptualize a variety of target groups and then determine, through formal or informal means, whether these groups are being reached. The purpose of conceptualizing target groups is to prevent us from assuming, perhaps wrongly, that the referrals to a program truly reflect the spectrum of young people in need of assistance.

Staff members can arrive at some general descriptions of target groups by using their own estimates derived from anecdotal reports of teachers, parents or community professionals. Another approach is to do a survey of adolescent drug abuse in the community. Such a survey is presented in "Sample Surveys of Drug Use Patterns" in the Appendix of *Alliance for Change* by James Crowley.

In the following paragraphs we offer one method of conceptualizing target groups; the target groups described are extrapolations from the data presented in Chapter Three. (So that we can see the forest for the trees, we have not repeated all of the studies cited in Chapter Three.) Readers should keep in mind that the target groups for their agencies or schools may differ somewhat, depending on the nature of the organization and the specific subgroup of young people served.

Heavy drug users

In a secondary-level school, 5% to 15% of the students are likely to be *daily* users of alcohol and/or other drugs. In a juvenile cor-

rections setting, 20% to 30% of offenders may be daily users of alcohol and 50% may be daily users of alcohol or marijuana. Between 15% and 25% of students in many schools can be called heavy users of alcohol and other drugs, i.e., they take more than one drug and use some chemicals three, four or more times per week. In a corrections setting, perhaps 75% of young offenders may be regular, although not necessarily daily, drug users.

Sex differences in heavy drug use

About twice as many boys as girls in the general student population use drugs daily. The incidence of binge drinking, i.e., having five or more consecutive drinks at least once during a two-week period, is about 50% for boys and 30% for girls.

Child abuse

It is difficult to make general statements about trends in physical abuse and neglect. Cohn (1983), who took into account a variety of factors, concluded that between 300,000 and 600,000 children are victims of physical or sexual abuse each year. Thus, the incidence of child abuse among school-age children is between 0.5% and 1.5%. Poverty is a factor in child abuse and among poor families the incidence of physical abuse is likely to be higher. In regard to sexual abuse, Gagnon (1965) reported that 26% of 1,200 college-age women had had some sexual experience with an adult before age 13. Another report (Kinsey, 1953) estimated that 20% to 24% of the women responding to a nationwide survey had been sexually molested as children.

Specific buildings and building complexes

In general, unless there are clear-cut reasons for some buildings to have abnormally high or low rates of intervention, the incidence of drug and alcohol problems in inner city, suburban and rural schools should be assumed to be no less than the averages specified previously. If the rate of intervention in one school building or building complex is far below the rates in other buildings or complexes, the discrepancy can probably be credited to the particular methods of early intervention used in the building, rather than to a true variation in the need for services. This, of course, can be a highly political situation, one that must be handled in the fashion that will most benefit students. For instance, it would be counterproductive to circulate a report saying that the principal of a particular school is doing a poor job.

Children of alcoholics

About 20% of the students in a given school may be affected by parental alcoholism or problem drinking. About 50% of heavy drug users have parents who are alcoholic or in some way are problem drug users. In a court population, the incidence of parental alcoholism can be more than 40%.

Athletes

Some parents and coaches tend to protect their promising young athletes for fear they will be kicked off the team or suffer other consequences. If no athletes or other star students are ever referred to a program, the situation should be reviewed to see if there are biases in the identification or internal referral process.

Methods for increasing identification

The number and types of young people identified in a program are functions of many variables: the level of staff awareness of both the problems and the early-intervention program; levels of staff trust in the program; degree of clear administrative support for the program; and other factors discussed in previous pages. These underlying factors should be evaluated periodically. The summary of effective, basic program components presented in Chapter Eleven should be useful in evaluating existing programs and planning new ones.

In this section we present a few techniques that some agencies and schools are using to identify youths with disruptive personal problems. These techniques will, of course, work differently in different schools or agencies. The decision of whether and how to use them is best left to the judgment of the early-intervention planning group.

Computer screening in the schools

The Princeton schools near Cincinnati, Ohio, have used a computer screening method to detect incipient problems in attendance, performance or general behavior. Short computer forms are sent out every two weeks to teachers, coaches and leaders of extracurricular activities. The forms contain questions about grades, academic performance, cooperation, involvement in class, deportment and attendance (see Figure 6-1). Besides having direct and immediate application to educational matters, the information gathered contributes to the early identification of drug or other personal problems.

Information on any current deficits in performance or behavior is referred to a counselor. Counselors know, then, every two or three weeks if any of the 300 students assigned each of them are having problems. Each school principal, who also receives a copy of the report, checks with counselors to see what action was taken with students manifesting problems.

The immediate feedback made possible by computer processing makes this method especially helpful in the process of early intervention. Information from many sources is collated quickly and given to a person who is in a position to help. The information is not very detailed or personal, but the system serves as a general "net" for identifying students with incipient problems. Parents of senior high school students receive quarterly reports; the junior high school has experimented with sending the biweekly reports home to parents.

Data entry for the 4,000 senior high school students takes about 20 hours. Of course, a great deal of time also went into the initial programming.

Use of outside consultants to stimulate interest

In the past few years, many schools have hired celebrities to discuss the issues of drug and alcohol abuse. While these celebrities do little to help the situation if there are no plans for a follow-up on the issues raised, they can be helpful if an early-intervention program is ready to accept referrals after their presentations. Counselors and schools with well-developed early-intervention programs have noted a marked increase in referrals after a celebrity has come to talk. Whether the celebrity is worth the price is another issue.

A more methodical, low-key and cost-effective way of doing the same thing is to hire local professionals from outside of the school district (it appears that this outsider position

helps) who are skilled at talking about a variety of issues of interest to children and adolescents. These professionals can talk to selected groups of students, small classes or 100 or 200 students at a time.

One outside consultant we know spends several days at the beginning of each school year discussing abusive relationships in families, problems of living with alcoholics, problems of personal drug use, self-assertion and other subjects. At the end of these talks, she passes out an assessment questionnaire (see Figure 6-2) that students fill out and return. Students are asked to indicate, on the form, their understanding of what a "support group" is and whether or not they would be interested in finding a specific type of support group or any other service. She then

STUDENT PERFORMANCE REPORT

TEACHER _____   WEEK OF _____

STUDENT'S NAME	I.D. NUMBER	COURSE CODE NUMBER	COURSE SECTION NUMBER	STATUS			COMMENTS (SEE CODE BELOW)					
				FAILING	BORDERLINE	WORKING BELOW EXPECTATION	1	2	3	4	5	6

COMMENTS CODE:
1 – Unprepared   2 – Incomplete Assignments   3 – Uncooperative   4 – Lack of Participation
5 – Violation of Classroom Rules   6 – Attendance Problems

Figure 6 – 1. Sample form for computer screening. This form would be used for general screening of all students, not for gathering information on specific students who are manifesting problems. It is brief, problem-oriented and easy for teachers to fill out.

confidentially contacts those students who indicate interest and invites them to attend a lecture about various support groups. Some students elect to join a school-sponsored group; others do not. Since this information is handled in confidence between the outside consultant and the students, only those students who agree to it have their names revealed to school staff members.

Presentations by local professionals have proved to be an effective way to motivate students to take the first step toward resolution of important personal issues. It is a useful way to start the school year and one or two such presentations every year would be a good option to consider in any school district.

Use of educational and outreach activities

When discussions on specific subjects like alcoholism in the family, personal drug use or child abuse are given in classrooms, it is not uncommon for students to come up after the class and ask more questions about the subject. Often these questions lead to a student requesting help with a problem related to that described in the presentation. Many young people are not so direct in requesting help, however. Some simply become negative about the topic being presented and hostile to the presenter. Others will show a marked change in activity—a normally subdued student becoming more active or a normally active student becoming quiet and withdrawn. These behavior changes during educational activities can be important tip-offs that a young person is in some kind of distress.

The identification of children of alcoholics is a natural and inevitable outgrowth of any drug intervention/prevention program. As the level of awareness of drug and alcohol problems increases and as more services are offered specifically for children of alcoholics,

---

ASSESSMENT QUESTIONNAIRE

(This questionnaire is confidential.)

1. My understanding of "support group" is: _____

    _____

    _____

    _____

    _____

2. I would be interested in a support group for:

    _____ Abusive relationships/families   _____ Self-confidence building

    _____ Children in chemically dependent   _____ Aftercare group for chemically dependent
           families   people
    _____ Learning to take risks and make friends   _____ All of the above topics

3. My name is: _____

4. My grade level is: _____

Figure 6 – 2. Sample assessment questionnaire. Confidential questionnaires can be an effective way of getting students to reach out for help.

these formerly "forgotten children" begin to receive help, as do students, probationers and social service clients whose problems result primarily from their own use of chemicals.

There are five common ways to reach children of alcoholics:

1. "Holding up the mirror" is a process of showing films and offering educational sessions about the plight of children of alcoholic parents. Children in need tend to reveal themselves to the person making the presentation during or after such sessions. This appears to be one of the most effective ways of getting them to identify themselves. One problem with relying too heavily on this method, however, is that it tends to reach the high achiever more than the underachiever or the person who acts out.

2. If it is known that a young person's parents are in treatment for alcoholism, she or he can be made aware of any services offered for children of alcoholics.

3. Sometimes a participant in an Alateen or concerned persons group recruits another person known to have an alcoholic parent.

4. Guidance counselors or other helping professionals sometimes refer clients to concerned persons groups when their problems appear to be related to parental alcoholism.

5. One method used often, but considered least effective is to advertise the group, listing its name, purpose, meeting time and referral information in a school or community publication.

Direct screening for children of alcoholics

Researchers and practitioners have found that asking direct questions about parental drinking problems is a very effective way to identify children of alcoholics. In studying clients of a teen medical and counseling clinic, Biek (1981) found that a simple two-part technique involving a written questionnaire and a semistructured interview proved very effective in screening. Clinic clients were asked, "Has the drinking of either parent created any problem for you?" This and a second question—"Have you known either of your parents to ever take a drink?"—were part of a written medical inventory used at the clinic. Those who answered "no" to the second question were not questioned further by an interviewer. All those who answered "yes" were asked if the drinking of either parent had ever created problems between the parents or with a close relative; if friends or relatives thought the parent had a drinking problem; and if the client had ever worried about the parent's drinking. These three variables had been identified by other researchers as being the most discriminating items for identifying children of parents with a drinking problem. Biek found that the written questions alone identified 14 (38%) of the 37 clients studied as being the children of parents with a drinking problem. Use of the semistructured interview increased this to 57%, a figure confirmed as accurate by further inquiry.

Initial Action

The ability to react appropriately to problem behaviors is crucial to early intervention. The key is for all concerned to know and accept their roles, do their jobs well and refrain from doing other people's jobs. Teachers, school administrators, parents, counselors, judicial and corrections personnel, concerned youth, and others must follow the specified procedures. Teachers, for example, must maintain high expectations for all students, let students know when their performance does not meet expected levels and make sure that parents are also aware of any problems. If interventions at this level do not help matters in short order, referral to administrative or counseling services should not be delayed.

While teachers, coaches, probation officers and others should be willing to discuss personal matters with young people, they can delay the early-intervention process if they try to solve problems all by themselves. It is just too difficult for any single person, no matter how intuitive or professionally competent, to make a clear determination about the nature of a young person's problems and the best course of action without seeing data from other sources. If teachers, coaches and others try to figure out what the problem is and what to do about it, they slow down the entire process of intervention with that young person, expend too much staff time, create a great deal of inconsistency throughout the system and decrease the likelihood that staff members will cooperate with implementation of the program.

This does not mean that teachers and coaches cannot be empathetic, caring and concerned. It does mean that they have to realize that regardless of their degree of skill as a counselor, which may or may not equal that of the early-intervention program staff, they are not in a position to bring a wide range of views into the picture. Consistency in all actions with young people has to be system-wide. If a young person has a sympathetic school nurse to go to with problems, he or she may be able to rest when hung over, avoid a class that may be particularly difficult and generally avoid the consequences of drug use. Similarly, if a student who is depressed or upset by family or other problems can receive just enough help to squeak by, despite pressure from other teachers, she or he may just make it through the school year. This pattern can repeat itself for three or four more years until the student graduates with minimal, but sufficient, effort and ends up in college, in military service or at a job, where pressures can build rapidly with less chance for help.

Three major types of referral

The word "referral" here means *referral to the early-intervention program*, not the re-

ferral from the program to community services.

According to some champions of the student assistance model, referrals should be based on performance and performance only. There are problems, however, with attempting to implement early-intervention programs solely on this basis. First, the highly intelligent and crafty students have no difficulty evading the system. Second, frequent breaks during the school year and the long summer break often interfere with the collection of information for performance evaluations. Because of the special situation in schools, the best way to reach and help the most young people in need of services is to allow for a variety of sources of and reasons for referrals. The spectrum should include referrals for drug violations, performance referrals, self-referrals and referrals from family members and friends.

Referrals related to violations of drug and alcohol regulations

As we have mentioned, the primary method of identification and referral in many programs is based on school disciplinary procedures. Again, this is a legitimate but limited approach, limited because it may give rise to a biased sample of students (primarily boys, primarily those who act out) and a negative image. The program as a whole may come to be viewed only as part of the disciplinary process and not as an independent helping service in its own right.

Performance referrals and referrals based on other classroom behaviors

Problems in attendance, academic performance and general classroom behavior are excellent *cues* for identifying drug users. Often, however, they are not sufficient to motivate or pressure students into taking action or cooperating with the actions taken by adults. After the performance cues are used to refer a student to a counselor, additional information obtained from the student, friends, family members and other teachers is crucial for developing a plan of action.

Schools have a slight advantage over the workplace in terms of performance standards. In school students are expected to work up to their potential. Thus, the amount of pressure that can be applied varies from student to student. In the workplace it is difficult to put pressure on employees who, regardless of their actual potential, meet the minimal standards of performance.

Self-referrals and referrals from family and friends

In some schools it is estimated that one third of the referrals are either self-referrals or referrals from family members and friends (see Chapter Nine). In other schools, it appears (but has not yet been documented) that not only are a great many referrals coming to the school counselors from the family but also that parents are starting to go directly to other sources in the community for help, partly as a result of the schools' or courts' early-intervention efforts. The keys to increasing such referrals are trust in the good will of the staff, belief that the services are helpful, the existence of a mutually agreed-on method of maintaining confidentiality and the visibility of the person or persons who represent the program.

If trust is high, even when the initial referral comes from a teacher or an administrator, the information that friends can provide can be very helpful. When a student is willing to cooperate, some counselors ask his or her permission to talk with friends and a great deal of useful information is thus obtained.

Overview of referral patterns

The actions and sequence of actions taken on behalf of a young person depend on the origin of the initial referral—in other words, on how she or he entered the system. Figure 6-3, "Program Flow for Performance Problems," details a sequence of actions for dealing with students who first come to staff attention because of behavioral or academic difficulties. For a self-referred student, the sequence differs somewhat; the counselor would probably interview the student first and then decide whether or not to solicit further information from other staff members.

When students enter the system for violating the rules on drug use and possession, a number of important decisions are often made before any of the preliminary assessment steps begin, depending on what disciplinary action is called for by school policies. Many schools, for instance, distinguish between first offenders and prior offenders in both discipline and assessment procedures. Often, first offenders are routed directly into some type of drug awareness or self-evaluation group or class, whereas those with prior violations face more stringent consequences.

Policies and procedures for dealing with drug use or possession violations are usually determined not by the early-intervention program staff but by school policy-making bodies, such as the school board. Schools vary in terms of how much emphasis they place on disciplinary procedures, but if these procedures prove counterproductive to early-intervention goals, every effort should be made to change them. For example, it is impossible to work students into any kind of intervention program if they are automatically expelled for a year after an infraction. Generally, automatic ten-day suspensions are also counterproductive. However, if students who face suspension are given the alternative of working with an early-intervention process, they can be hooked into the helping system much more smoothly.

The following procedures constitute one school's policy for dealing with drug possession or use:

1. The student's parents attend a conference with the assistant principal.

2. The student is suspended for one day.

3. The parents must choose by a specified date, *one* of the following options:

PROGRAM FLOW FOR PERFORMANCE PROBLEMS

Student Behavior or Performance Problem

↓

CONCERNED STAFF MEMBER

- notes problem behavior pattern
- shares concern with the student
- specifies expected standards of achievement or behavior

↓

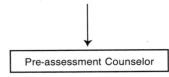

If no change in behavior/performance

- discusses situation with student again
- tells him/her of the need for action
- discusses case with early-intervention program counselor
- refers the student to counselor (if no change)

↓

Pre-assessment Counselor

performs some or all of the following:

- sends out Behavioral Observation Report Form to all concerned
- consults with teachers, counselors, administrators, others
- sets up conference with concerned teacher and student
- develops behavior/performance profile
- interviews student
- meets with parents to inform and to get data
- considers appropriateness of referral to assessment team

↓

Assessment and Referral Team

- reviews student profile from pre-assessment counselor
- develops total profile from performance/behavior data
- considers referral options
- develops action plan and behavior contract
- refers to appropriate services in the school or community
- assigns responsibility to monitor student's performance and specifies a follow-up date

Figure 6 – 3. Program flow chart for performance problems.

a. a chemical assessment by the county assessment agency,

b. an assessment by an approved private hospital (specified by the school),

c. individual sessions with a chemical health specialist, or

d. participation in an education/awareness/personal assessment group.

Given this range of options, the student and parents almost always choose the chemical health specialist. If they do not choose one of the options and complete the appropriate steps by a certain date, the procedures become more stringent. This automatic sequence of choices for a first offense can be helpful to the early-intervention program coordinator whose time is severely limited. Parent conferences must take place soon after the incident and are often difficult to schedule, especially by an early-intervention program counselor who is already involved in group facilitation or inservice training. The automatic process of the first several steps in early intervention allows a counselor to meet with the student and parents after the emergency pressures have abated.

In referrals based on academic performance or classroom behavior problems, the process typically proceeds more methodically. A counselor usually attempts to clarify the situation with the referring staff member and, if there seems to be little basis for the referral, the process may stop there. If investigation seems warranted, data are then requested from other teachers, who complete written forms to be returned within a specified time. It is best if such forms do not carry an inherent bias either by their design (e.g., questions about specific drug-related behaviors) or by their source (i.e., the "drug program"). Unbiased forms from an unbiased source, such as the student guidance bureau, work best in the earliest stages of intervention.

Patterns of referrals from staff members

Experience shows that a small percentage of school staff members make most of the referrals. In most schools with active early-intervention programs, between 10% and 20% of the staff members actively refer regularly, while the majority are cooperative but somewhat less active. About 5% to 10% tend to be hostile to the program. Since it is likely that any program will have a small core of actively referring teachers, it is important to ensure that this group includes people from strategic areas in the building. For example, if all of the shop teachers and none of the English teachers are enthusiastic about the program, it may be necessary for program staff members to devote extra time and ingenuity to get some of the latter involved. This kind of focused outreach can range from one-to-one conversations to special inservice training.

Front-line staff members, such as teachers, make referrals on the basis of attendance and performance problems, disruptive behavior, obvious physical changes and other concrete cues. Some, naturally, are more closely attuned than others and more able to read subtle signs of trouble in students' classroom behaviors. And there are always a few empathetic, emotionally attuned staff members who pick up intuitive, "gut level" cues with a high degree of accuracy.

Staff inservice training and community outreach are crucial. When staff members understand how difficulties with certain students may be related to drug abuse, drug dependency, parental alcohol use and other family problems, and when they know that helpful services are available, referrals from all sources increase.

Why some staff members do not refer

One significant barrier to initial action can be the attitudes and feelings of school staff members. The following summary of typical barriers, some of which have already been mentioned, can serve as a useful guideline for inservice training:

○ Many teachers who do not make referrals tend to see students who use drugs or those who act out as "lost causes." Sometimes these teachers or other staff members fall victim to the "good kids vs. bad kids" syndrome and believe it is best to just let the bad kids go in favor of helping the good kids.

○ When parents do not cooperate in the early-intervention process, some staff members tend to ignore their students until their behavior is egregious. They come to believe that unless things really get out of hand, these kids are not worth the trouble because only the most obvious behavior will convince their parents to take action.

○ As we have noted, some teachers prefer to counsel students, while others fear that they will get young people into trouble if they make referrals.

○ Some staff members do not want to be "the heavy" or get a reputation for being confrontive. They fear losing their rapport with young people.

○ Sometimes fear of physical reprisals or vandalism against those who confront students on drug use inhibits referrals.

○ Occasionally school administrators have not made it clear that cooperation with the early-intervention program is a job requirement, that staff must refer students when procedures call for it. When administrators are willing to take a clear stand on the issue, referrals from all areas of the school usually increase markedly.

○ Personal issues can also be a factor in the referral process. Just as counselors and therapists must work out their own issues with their family members to be effective in their professional roles, so too must teachers and coaches. Their family histories affect their roles in the early-intervention process. Alcohol and drug abuse is a very personal issue for many people. It is surprising how many of our friends and associates have had alcohol problems in their families. Many of these people are successful and productive, but still have some attitudes or biases about these problems.

One program coordinator told us about a teacher who spent months counseling his students about their family problems rather than referring them for appropriate help. When the teacher discussed this with the program coordinator, he started to realize that he did not know who he was unless he was in the middle of some conflict. Through a training program, he came to realize that his mother, who was alcoholic, had greatly influenced his adult behavior. He still tended to take care of his younger brothers and sisters and negotiated most family arguments.

"In case after case where we found overinvolved and overextended teachers," said one counselor, "we found people who had never resolved their own issues related to alcohol problems in the family of origin. They were meeting their own needs by making themselves constantly available to the kids. These teachers, although trying to be helpful, have a great need to keep the kids where they are rather than helping them improve."

In every school or agency, there will also be adults who have their own problems with alcohol or other drugs. Such people are sometimes uncooperative with or hostile to early-intervention programs.

Not all referrals will be appropriate

Some staff members are overly zealous in referring young people for help. Adults who have undergone treatment themselves or who have been through training on chemical abuse problems, for example, sometimes overreact and start seeing drug problems where there are none. This phenomenon is a natural response to the training process; with appropriate feedback, an overly zealous staff member can become a fine source of appropriate referrals. An overenthusiastic eagerness to help young people is, after all, a much more positive state of affairs than the inertia and apathy exhibited by those who do not think they can help at all.

Sometimes staff members are hostile to a program. They may have a good reason if, for instance, an early-intervention program staff member did not act in a competent manner in the past. It is helpful to convince these people to talk to the early-intervention program staff. Some teachers have come in to early-intervention programs and said, "I wouldn't refer a kid to you if it was the last place on earth. I don't trust you, I don't think you like kids, and I think you're out to get them." It is important that these teachers say these things to the core team because they certainly are saying them to others in the school. Usually, part of what they have to report will be valid but exaggerated. These teachers must be heard, and the validity of their concerns must be considered, but they should also be confronted if they are acting inappropriately. Administrative backup is important if a teacher is, in fact, making inappropriate comments and taking disruptive actions.

Feedback to teachers is essential

Staff members who refer students to the program need constant feedback as to the appropriateness or inappropriateness of their actions. They should be made generally aware of what has happened to the student as a result of the referral and of any positive changes effected by his or her involvement in the program. Keep in mind that groups and drug awareness classes rarely bring about instantaneous transformations; teachers and other front-line staff members may not see any immediate radical improvement in classroom performance. When a young person is making progress, the teacher or coach who was concerned enough to make the referral should be told that it may have done a great deal to help. A simple form, such as the one in Figure 6-4, is an efficient way to provide this feedback.

Student involvement in faculty inservice programs can be very helpful in developing staff support for a program. When students tell faculty members about the program's impact on them, they usually have a strong, positive effect on those who are reluctant to devote any time or energy to the early-intervention program.

Special programs

Many schools today host a variety of special programs geared toward meeting the intellectual, emotional and physical needs of students. Here we consider two important categories of special programs: the childcare or child-study teams and the "alternative school" programs. Both can have a strong influence on the conduct of the early-intervention process in a given building.

Child-study teams

Most schools in the country are mandated, through a variety of federal programs, to provide a team of selected staff members to deal with "special needs students." These teams usually include a social worker, a learning-disabilities teacher, a school psychologist, appropriate guidance staff members and, perhaps, a school administrator. They are charged with screening and assessing students who have general learning disabilities; special learning disabilities; special learning and behavioral problems; or behavior management problems.

Child-study teams are very important in the identification of young people who may be in need of services for drug abuse or other personal problems. Many treatment center staffs report that their clients seem to have more learning disabilities than other students. It is hypothesized, then, that students with special learning disabilities or behavioral problems are at greater risk for drug use and serious drug-related problems. Whether or not this hypothesis is true, it is important that a representative from the early-intervention program be a member of this team to integrate the early-intervention program with other services and to educate other staff members about the possibility of drug problems. Also, all members of the special child-study team should be given an opportunity to undergo intensive training regarding the problem of adolescent alcohol and drug abuse.

"Alternative school" programs

Many school districts offer "alternative high schools," "mini-schools," "work release programs," "storefront schools" or abbreviated schedules. In many school districts, these programs serve students who have been moved out of the normal system because of behavioral problems and inability to work in the regular classroom setting. These programs play an important role in the education of the students involved and we have no overall comment about their positive or negative effects. There are, however, three factors to consider in relation to early intervention:

o Students in special programs may not be pressured to perform as well as students in other programs. For those who are on drugs, such enabling may allow them to stay stuck with their drug problems. It is likely that some of the young people in alternative school programs are there *because* of performance deficits related to drug problems.

o Alternative school programs are excellent places to identify drug problems. In many schools, the staff members of these programs have been very eager, willing participants in training regarding adolescent drug issues.

o Sometimes a political issue arises regarding the amount of time that the early-intervention program staff can devote to the alternative school program. If the students in the alternative school program are labeled bad kids, the type of administrative support needed for in-depth work in this area may be difficult to elicit.

To: Date:

From:

This is to update you on information regarding

_____

Since the referral to me for service:

_____ I have contacted the student and the home to begin my assessment.

_____ I have completed the assessment and a referral for service is being made.

_____ The services have begun and he/she will be out of school for a period of time.

_____ The student has been placed in a support group.

_____ I have completed an assessment and there appears to be no major problem.

_____ Other

_____

Please call me if you have any questions.   Phone #: _____

Figure 6 – 4. Sample of a form by which program staff members can give teachers feedback on the referrals they make.

Next we discuss the sources of data; the relative importance of different types of data; the use of a student identification number in program records; and a basic data-gathering form.

Data Gathering

Once an adolescent is identified as having a problem that has not been resolved through normal academic or disciplinary procedures, the next step is to do a preliminary assessment to determine whether drugs or other personal problems are causing the difficulty. This step begins with the gathering of information about the young person and culminates in a judgment about the nature of the problem. The specific techniques used to weigh various factors in the assessment of adolescent drug abuse and related problems are too complex to be covered here. A detailed treatment of the subject awaits another volume. Nonetheless, the early-intervention program itself is structured to facilitate assessment. The whole point of incremental intervention is to methodically walk young people through successive levels of intervention. The basic concepts and premises presented in preceding chapters, if discussed and clarified within a given school or agency, can help make the assessment process much smoother.

Sources and types of information

Many sources of information have a bearing on how a student benefits from an early-intervention program. These include data about the original drug-related offense, if there was one; teachers' comments about academic performance and classroom behavior; cumulative records on the student; information volunteered by the student; and reports from parents, friends and other concerned persons. Social service agencies sometimes have a great deal on family background to offer, and probation officers have data on legal problems.

Before beginning a search of the various sources of information, most program counselors review their own memory files, asking such questions as "How many times have I heard this name before? Have I heard about his parents? Have I heard other kids refer to him as a 'drug user' or as a kid whose parents treat him rough? Have I heard parents of some of the other kids I deal with mention this student? Have I heard he was one of the students having trouble in the junior high school? Has he been chronically absent from school? Did I ever see him hanging out in the parking lot or any other place where drug use is likely to occur?"

None of these questions is diagnostic and none can be used to confront a student. Hearsay information can be useful if the reliability of the source is known, but it is neither fair nor appropriate to make decisions based on such information without confirmation. However, it does help us answer questions about how much research is needed, how deep we have to dig and how fast we should move.

Some considerations for the implications of the various sources and types of information follow.

Data on the original drug violation

It is important to know all of the circumstances surrounding the drug violation and how typical this behavior is for the student. It is helpful to know whether this incident was one of the first times she or he had used drugs and whether it was a very positive, neutral or negative experience.

School records

School records are good sources of information on past behavior up to the most recent reporting period. If drug use is a problem, records are likely to show changes in the degree, although not necessarily in kinds, of problems. Students whose academic performance declines in response to drug use often already have some problems in academic performance. Then there are those students who do excellent work that deteriorates rap-

Can Sources of Data Be Kept Confidential?

One question that arises regarding data gathering and interviews is whether or not the sources of data should be revealed to the young person. Each counselor must have a clear understanding of all regulations relevant to this issue but must be allowed some flexibility in dealing with individual cases. We interviewed counselors about their approaches to this issue and present here a summary of our findings.

All counselors agreed that the sources of data directly related to a disciplinary action or an action in which the school takes a strong positive stance (such as referral to a hospital for medical or psychiatric emergencies) must always be revealed, preferably in writing.

The most common general "policy" of counselors is that they try to avoid making the specific sources of data an issue, especially if a number of

sources have revealed similar behaviors. They try to steer clear of this issue, at first, because students are likely to be defensive and engage in personality disputes rather than deal with their own behavioral patterns.

One counselor told us, "I'll probably tell a student how many teachers have expressed concern, but I won't tell him or her who exactly did so unless the teacher has given me specific permission."

Another counselor expressed how she handles the situation: "If I feel there is a problem lying ahead with convincing the student or parents about a drug issue, I ask the teacher's permission to share the source of my data if it becomes necessary. I do that as a regular practice, but I don't usually have to name all the specific sources of my information. Once the student relaxes with me, it becomes less of an issue. When I have an athlete, however, I try to get as many people as possible involved in the data-gathering process, people who

are willing to share information face-to-face with the kid and the parent. Often there is a lot of denial among parents of athletes and we need to go over our data point by point."

There are counselors, however, who refuse to get into the bind of not being allowed to reveal the sources of the data. One counselor said, "When I accept a referral without the kid knowing the source of the concern, I spend too much time arguing about his or her anger over it. The student wants to figure out just who the concerned teachers were. I insist that teachers let me reveal my sources of information."

How well the program is accepted and trusted by staff members is a determinant in how willing individuals are to confront students directly. In-service training about the goals and procedures of the program can help matters immensely. Teachers have to be willing to take some risks, and they will if they believe those risks are worth it. They need to know they will be backed up by the program staff or the administration, not because they are always right but because they are sincere and concerned.

idly when personal problems arise in their lives. In general, cumulative records can show useful information about grades, extra-curricular activities and disciplinary problems. They show the "base rate," or the general potential shown by the student in the past, rather than current information. Since action on drug problems may be called for before the end of a semester, before general data are reported and recorded, it may be necessary to obtain a more current update by asking teachers about current performance.

Individual class attendance reports

These reports can be useful in ascertaining patterns of truancy that may be related to drug use or other disruptive personal problems.

Data reported from teachers and other school staff members

Although such information should not be relied on to determine the nature of a problem, it can be of significance in defining its extent. Teachers can certainly report specific behaviors, trouble signs and their perceptions about the likely causes, but they should not be asked to diagnose the problem. The relative weighting of causal factors need not be done by front-line staff members.

Interview with the student

An interview can be of greater or lesser importance, depending on the specific student and the particular goals of the interview. Sometimes an interview can be a very important source of new information. At other times its primary purpose is to make the student aware of the situation and to check his or her general attitude about recent events (more about this in Chapter Seven).

Data from the parents

Concrete information from parents can help staff members fill out a picture of a student's behavior. For example, parents may verify that a student has a new group of friends or is staying out late and disobeying home rules. Another important, but more diffuse kind of information can be gained from observing parents' reactions to situations; their ways of protecting or not protecting their children; and their degree of interest in the problem.

It is a good policy to consider all sources of information in every case. For instance, one drug awareness program counselor told us that she does not rely heavily on cumulative records because any important data will already be known to the student's assigned counselor. However, she told of one case in which she could not find any clear explanation for a student's poor performance during an interview. When she looked at the cumulative file she discovered that the student's mother had died less than a year before and that, for some reason, her death had not been reported to the counselor and the student had not mentioned it. The mother's death and related unresolved issues surrounding her demise were the probable cause of the young person's depression and, in turn, poor performance.

Having proved useful in screening the general student population for disruptive personal problems, computers are also improving the data-gathering process in some early-intervention programs. If the general information system of the school is computerized and the information on student attendance and performance is relevant and up-to-date, program coordinators should definitely consider making use of this resource. The ideal situation, of course, is for the needs of the early-intervention program to be integrated into the system from the beginning, when computerized data management is being developed for the school. The early-intervention program staff should not pass up an opportunity to be involved in the planning stages of a computerized information system. Backtracking at a later date is more difficult and time-consuming and usually yields less satisfactory results.

A basic data-gathering form

Some drug intervention programs use highly detailed data-gathering forms that require

—— BEHAVIORAL OBSERVATION REPORT ——

Concerning:

(Detach this portion before you return the form)

Student I.D. No.

BEHAVIORAL OBSERVATION REPORT

This is a CONFIDENTIAL document and may be used only for the purpose of assessing potential behavioral problems of the student named above. This form should be kept in a secure place and the discussion of its contents outside of the professional scope of the educator is to be avoided. The fact that you have received this request for information should not be considered an indication of the presence of problems for this particular student.

ATTENDANCE: Have you noticed any problems regarding this student's attendance in your class or extracurricular activity (actual absenteeism, documented truancy, tardiness, frequent schedule changes for your class, request for passes to leave the room, etc.)? **YES** ☐ **NO** ☐ If yes, give dates and times, if possible.

ACADEMIC PERFORMANCE: Has this student's academic performance changed noticeably from a previous level of functioning? **YES** ☐ **NO** ☐ If yes, please note what changes have occurred and when they happened or began to happen.

Is this student currently failing your class or performing markedly below potential? **YES** ☐ **NO** ☐

ATTITUDES AND BEHAVIORS: Have this student's attitudes towards school or towards your class or extracurricular activity changed markedly? **YES** ☐ **NO** ☐ If yes, in what way?

Has this student shown any signs of increased apathy, withdrawal, drowsiness or other indications of decreased energy? **YES** ☐ **NO** ☐ Comments:

Has this student been acting-out more in your class or extracurricular activity; shown signs of increased activity level; been more argumentative or generally fidgety and agitated? **YES** ☐ **NO** ☐ Comments:

SOCIAL BEHAVIOR: Have you noticed any marked change in the friends with whom this student associates? **YES** ☐ **NO** ☐ Comments:

CHEMICALS: Have you had any concerns about this student's use of alcohol or other drugs? **YES** ☐ **NO** ☐ Comments:

STRENGTHS: What do you see as this student's strengths?

WEAKNESSES: What do you see as this student's weaknesses?

***   ***   ***

Have you shared with the student any concerns about the issues mentioned above or any other aspect of this student's behavior? **YES** ☐ **NO** ☐ Comments:

Do you have information that you would prefer to discuss with a counselor face-to-face? **YES** ☐ **NO** ☐ Comments:

What time and place is best for you?

Would you be willing to be involved in a conference with this student? **YES** ☐ **NO** ☐
With the student and the parents? **YES** ☐ **NO** ☐

Name _____ Date _____

Please detach the student's name from the top of this form, fold it and return to:

Figure 6–5. Behavioral Observation Report. The best data-gathering forms are structured by categories of behavior and thus relatively simple to fill out.

staff members to enumerate the number of times a student has bloodshot eyes or liquor on the breath and to supply information on family relations and job performance. This type of comprehensive form annoys teachers because of the amount and types of questions asked. In addition to asking for information that does not routinely concern teachers, it has built-in biases not appropriate to early stages of intervention.

At the other end of the spectrum is the completely open-ended form that provides no guidelines at all. Teachers in a hurry are unlikely to have either the time or the patience to sit down and formulate behavior categories to consider for a student who is having problems.

Data-gathering forms should be relatively simple, structured around behavior categories and unbiased, both in terms of design and source. We suggest that a simple behavioral observation form, such as that in Figure 6-5, be used. It provides several categories to consider but is still open-ended enough so that it will not slant responses. The option of simply answering "yes" or "no" allows respondents to at least give their impressions if they do not have time to write comments. Some forms carry this option further by including a checklist under each major behavior category. All the teacher or other staff person has to do is check off particular problems.

The "strengths and weaknesses" section of the form may seem irrelevant, yet it has proved very helpful. It encourages teachers who may have been angry and frustrated with a given student to step back and consider positive aspects of her or his character or habits. Even such comments as "very social," "polite" and "dresses nicely" can help break down a student's initial resistance when first talking to a counselor. Students are often surprised to hear that teachers recognize strengths in them; this positive feedback can facilitate the intervention process in subtle ways.

The source of the request for information

should not build too great a bias into a teacher's or coach's perceptions. Some early-intervention programs avoid biasing responses by using the same forms used by the administration, the guidance office or childcare teams; in many schools, these are called grade and attitude forms or status reports. Nonetheless, the source of the request has a legitimate bearing on what information is reported. Comments submitted to an assistant principal may, for example, be restricted to concrete, observable facts, whereas those sent to a student assistance counselor may include personal hunches. The name of the person to whom the report should be returned should, therefore, be clearly marked on the outside of the form.

A simple statement about the confidentiality of the information serves as a good reminder to the staff. The issue of confidentiality is, of course, covered in all inservice training sessions but is important enough to warrant a reminder on the form.

Student identification numbers

Students' identities can be protected by the use of identification numbers unique to the early-intervention system. The reasons for this are that behavioral report forms may end up in the wrong office by accident, or the forms may be reviewed by outside staff as part of research or program evaluation projects.

Identification numbers can be assigned either when request forms are sent out or when a student is interviewed by a program staff member. The student's name and number should be recorded on a small index card and filed in a secure location. The only people who should have access to this information are those who are part of the early-intervention program. Student information forms, on which are compiled all information gathered from various sources, should include only this number, not the name. If data lead to no immediate conclusions and no action is taken, these forms can be filed for review af-

"Not With a Bang But a Whimper"

In his poem *The Hollow Men*, T. S. Eliot wrote: "This is the way the world ends, not with a bang but a whimper." Although early-intervention programs do not pretend to such a global perspective, there is a lesson here for all of us.

Many people believe the success or failure of early-intervention programs wholly depends on the ideology they espouse. Thus, someone who believes drug addiction is a disease may feel that belief in that concept alone is bound to lead to effective programming. Others may feel that recognizing drug abuse as a moral problem, a conditioned reflex or a Communist plot will automatically lead to appropriate action.

While there is much to be said for the ability of great ideas to be the prime movers or changers of social conditions, the real world is often affected more by the accumulation of small actions or inactions than by great ideas. Many programs fail because the first meetings were too unfocused or the publicity was so poor that no one came. Or perhaps the ideas were good, but they were presented to the wrong people. Or perhaps the chairman of the committee just did not know how to advance beyond the talking stage. Or perhaps the meetings were excellent but no decisions were made at the end of the meetings and no deadlines for completion of the tasks were set ....

When people never become focused, when decisions are never made, when differences are never resolved, frustration builds and people give up. The programs that are successful select relevant, realistic goals and pursue the achievement of those goals to the last detail. The issue of adolescent drug use has to be considered in program planning but there are limitations to this issue alone. Of equal importance are the issues of teamwork and organizational dynamics.

ter a specified period. If later review shows no need for further action, the information can either be eliminated or filed to await another review.

Confidentiality

Confidentiality is an ethical and professional issue as well as a legal one. School policies must, of course, be compatible with existing laws, but a preoccupation with the legal aspect of this issue can be both misleading and counterproductive. James Crowley outlines a balanced approach to the confidentiality issue in his book *Alliance for Change*. (See the Appendix for an excerpt and adaptation of his discussion of these confidentiality issues.)

***   ***   ***

Simply by providing services for identification, initial action and data gathering, a school or agency is contributing a great deal to the early-intervention process. Then, if competent, cooperative assessment counselors from the community are readily available, the data can be interpreted and decisions can be made with no missed steps, dropped balls or unnecessary delays. Whether or not outside consultants are available is, however, almost always a matter of some concern. Most schools and court services that are serious about early intervention have taken upon themselves the responsibility of developing a certain number of basic services. These will be described in the next chapter.

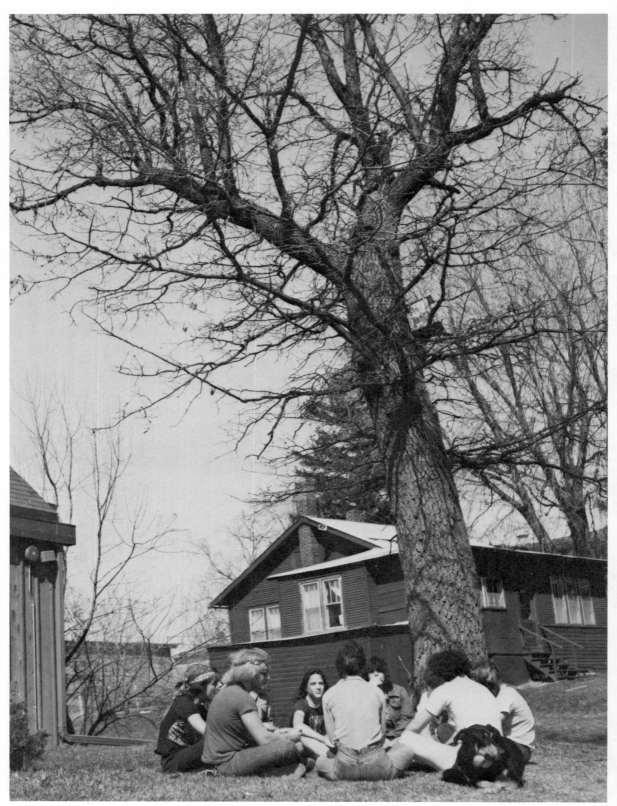

photo: Joseph Muldoon

CHAPTER SEVEN

BASIC IN-HOUSE SERVICES
Pre-assessment and Groups

Early intervention is sometimes seen as a process of informally screening the youth population for general problems and referring those with apparent problems to appropriate community resources. "Keep it simple," an advocate of such a model would say. "If a kid seems to have a problem, check him out, and send him to a counselor in the community if he needs help."

The trouble is, it is not as simple as it sounds. "Checking a kid out" summarizes a host of details about what does and does not constitute a drug problem; what intuitive skills a school counselor may or may not have; what definition of adequate service should be adopted; and how the effectiveness of both the screening process and the agency in the community can be verified.

Since almost all adolescents experiment with mood-altering chemicals and the majority use at least monthly, we have a very large group of drug users who need a wide variety of interventions. Most young drug users will not need an assessment by a professional agency outside the schools or the courts. Even if a young person does need such an assessment, there are no omniscient assessment authorities who, on their own and in a short time, can tell people in the schools and the courts much that is not already known. If those who refer young people for assessment do a thorough job of gathering data and contributing to the assessment process, however, their efforts, in combination with the clinical skills of a professional assessment counselor, can make the whole greater than the sum of its parts.

Furthermore, most young people identified as having incipient problems are not so destructive in their behavior or delinquent in their responsibilities that they can be forced to do anything about their problems. Unless some services are readily available in the schools, these kids may not get the assistance they need until they are deeply in trouble.

For a variety of reasons, then, early-intervention programs can benefit by offering some low-level intervention services to young people. By "low level," we mean inexpensive, not time-consuming and not personally intrusive. In this chapter we describe three general areas of service that can be of greatest benefit: services related to preliminary assessment; services for referral to and coordination with community agencies; and support services for young people who are attempting to refrain from drug use.

Preliminary Assessment Services

The goal of preliminary assessment is to gather the information needed to make a decision about what should be done next in the early-intervention process. Since the point of the process is to take action, it is usually not necessary to compile a complete analysis of the young person's family, a thorough evaluation of personal strengths and weaknesses or a complete drug history. Some preliminary assessments may only involve reviewing the information presented on paper, perhaps clarifying it in an interview with the young person and screening out the referral as inappropriate.

Early-intervention programs must be prepared to maintain several assessment-related services: interviewing young people and parents; monitoring behavior, if necessary, until clearer patterns emerge; sponsoring Insight Groups and making use of the information gained therein; referring youths for assessments by service providers in the community; and cooperating with those agencies to help implement their recommendations.

By offering these preliminary assessment services, schools can avoid false alarms and focus more closely on those students who most need our help. If we can identify those who use drugs but do not have critical drug problems and engage them in low-level interventions, we can reserve the more intense services of an outside agency for those who appear to have more serious problems.

Pre-assessment interviews

As has already been made clear by our review of data-gathering systems, the face-to-face interview plays an important role, but not the *only* role, in learning about a young person's problems, strengths and weaknesses. However, an interview can do much more than simply provide new data. Some important reasons for meeting face-to-face with a young person include:

- *To offer personal support.* Perhaps the person has not had anyone to talk to about the present situation. An expression of personal concern by the interviewer can be a very important part of the process.
- *To ensure that the person is fully aware of the situation.* We cannot *presume* that a young person really understands the nature or seriousness of the current situation, the specific impending consequences and the various options available. The face-to-face interview is the only way to guarantee that such matters are understood.
- *To learn the young person's viewpoint.* An interview may be necessary to find out what the person thinks about the situation: In his or her opinion, are the data being presented valid? Are they fair? Is he or she being singled out? Is the person actually glad to be getting the attention?
- *To assess the level of concern.* The interviewer should try to gauge how invested the person is in working on whatever problem is being faced.
- *To assess the level of control.* Is the person willing and able to take control of the situation? For instance, will she or he agree to a contract to abstain from chemicals? Does she or he appear to be the type who will honor commitments?
- *To gather new data.* Again, this is not the only reason for doing an interview, but the revelation of new data is sometimes a very important aspect of the interview.
- *To gain some general impressions.* A personal interview provides many visual and emotional clues, such as physical appearance, style of dress and alertness or lack of alertness.

The goals of a particular interview vary from program to program, from counselor to counselor, from case to case. Some counselors who work in schools with punitive disciplinary procedures frequently find it necessary to give students support and hope. In informal programs without comprehensive methods of gathering data, interviewers may have to spend a great deal of time trying to uncover specific information, whereas in programs with more comprehensive data-gathering services, interviewers are free to focus on other issues.

The process of interviewing is covered in hundreds of publications. One particularly helpful book that addresses this subject with due consideration given to the goals of specific interviewing or counseling situations is Gerard Egan's *The Skilled Helper*.

Monitoring

Patience is a key word for adults working with young people during the early stages of intervention. Assessment of adolescent drug problems is rarely a cut-and-dried process. Rather, it often entails monitoring the young person for a time to see what patterns emerge. Parents, concerned staff members and the drug user explore what the drug user knows and feels, and how she or he lives, relates to others and reacts to new information, new experiences and new relationships.

This ability to monitor ongoing behavior differentiates early-intervention programs from outside assessment services in the community. It is one of the greatest strengths of the early-intervention program. As one counselor put it, "Evaluation as an ongoing process is far more applicable to adolescents than to adults. If you're not looking at them over time, you're not doing them justice."

An ongoing monitoring process is frequently used in schools when a student *appears* to have some problems with chemicals or other issues, but the picture is not yet clear enough for definite action. Often, members of a school program's core team meet and review a number of cases being monitored to see if any problems have reemerged since the original incident that brought a young person to the attention of the early-intervention program staff. Probation officers and professionals in community agencies also participate in this type of ongoing monitoring process, but they are at a disadvantage. Only schools are in a position to monitor very closely—on a daily basis if need be—how well particular students are living up to their responsibilities.

Ongoing monitoring should not be seen as a way to procrastinate or avoid issues. It is a legitimate and effective option. The key to its success is to not allow it to become haphazard and disorganized to the point where staff members lose track of those youths they have been monitoring over time.

A group approach to pre-assessment

Another preliminary assessment service is the Insight Group. Although adults do have legitimate power over children and adolescents, the way that people relate to drugs is ultimately, at least when they reach adulthood, their own decision. Early-intervention programs, while insisting on abstinence for students in high school, do well to give those young people the information and experiences needed to help them make decisions, in both the immediate and the distant future.

A group setting can facilitate attempts to help young people increase their knowledge about drugs and their awareness of how their lives are being affected by drug use. Some advantages of the group approach are:

o The imparting of information is more productive. The examples volunteered by participants add to and clarify the material offered by a presenter; the questions asked by each individual member and the reactions of other members contribute to the entire group learning experience.

o When individuals are trying to increase their awareness of drug problems and the negative effects that drugs have had on their own lives, group members can share their observations.

o When a person's defenses are high, peer confrontation can be invaluable in breaking through those barriers.

Insight Groups are one useful method of meeting the basic goals of imparting knowledge and awareness about drug problems to young people who are already involved with drugs. The term "Insight Group" was coined by Jim Crowley in 1977, when he began developing this model. In using the term here, we mean a structured series of didactic presentations, group discussions and, sometimes, confrontations concerning the use and abuse of drugs. Schools, court services and social service agencies can offer these groups. When offered in a school setting, they are sometimes called Insight Classes.

The Insight Group model

Insight Groups are often the first formal in-house intervention services initiated by schools or court systems. Insight Groups are part class and part interactive group. In some systems they are used almost automatically whenever a young person is discovered in possession or under the influence of a mood-altering chemical. Although many of the techniques used in Insight Groups and other drug awareness groups may be similar, the unique population from which the group members are drawn—those whose drug use has come to the attention of adults in authority—gives Insight Groups a dynamic very different from that of groups representative of the general population of young people.

Insight Groups are not open-ended. A specific number of sessions are offered. (A nine-session program is described in detail in Appendix A.) Clear guidelines are established regarding abstinence from chemicals, attendance requirements and participation. In some systems participants are even given "assignment books" that contain a variety of written self-evaluation exercises to be completed before sessions begin. In other systems the printed material used in the groups is kept to a minimum but the structure is still quite tight.

The structure of Insight Groups provides guidelines for neophyte facilitators and gives experienced facilitators ample opportunity to utilize advanced group skills. The structure also assures that the young people involved will be given an opportunity to acquire information and to assess their own drug use. Participants work on personal issues within a clearly defined framework. Those with less severe problems and more ability to take advantage of the opportunity will derive benefits, while those who are more weighed down by drug and/or other personal problems may not cooperate enough to get much out of the process. A person's ability to benefit from the process itself is, therefore, a method of behavioral assessment.

No matter how young persons enter a group—voluntarily or due to academic or behavioral problems—they follow the same course through the Insight process. They will usually sign a contract not to use drugs; they agree to a counseling session of some sort with their parents; and they know that during or immediately after the nine Insight sessions they will meet individually with a counselor in order to clarify issues, share personal information and, perhaps, ask for more help. A 30-day follow-up session with a counselor is usually scheduled as well. How, where, when and who is involved in these other activities depend on specific school or court procedures.

Group composition

Some schools and agencies use Insight Groups as an alternative to suspension or other disciplinary actions. When caught while intoxicated or in possession of alcohol or other drugs, instead of being expelled or incarcerated immediately, a young person may be sent to an Insight Group. Such Insight Groups tend, then, to involve only "hard bust" kids who have been caught red-handed. If this is the sole criterion used for inclusion, the groups tend to take on the complexion of being for "tough" kids. A heterogeneous group provides more balance. This has at least two benefits: First, the involvement of different types of youths helps to moderate group dynamics. For instance, the more thoughtful, restrained members do not feed into the antisocial (or, more likely, anti-adult) pronouncements of the acting-out types; the more outgoing ones help draw out the shy members. Second, the group does not acquire an image in the school as being exclusively or primarily for one type of drug user.

It is extremely important not to confuse the function of an Insight Group with that of an abstinence support group. Some schools and agencies have thought it beneficial to place youths who are trying to stay drug-free and newly identified drug users in the same groups. However, those who are being confronted with their drug use problems for the first time are usually angry and resistant to change. They may take their anger out on the young people who are trying to remain drug-free. This is an unfair burden to place on the latter; they should have their own support group with others who have already decided that it is in their own best interest to stay away from drugs.

Goals of Insight Groups

The first goal of Insight Groups is *assessment*. Participants may not share feelings or make significant changes while in the group, but if the group can make the participants, the counselor, school administrators and their parents aware of the nature and scope of their problems, the effort has been worthwhile. By the end of the group, facilitators should understand each member's specific pattern of drug use and the impact that drugs have had on each member's life. Participants not only should be able to name the consequences of their drug use but also should have some feeling-level awareness of its effects on their lives. Other important goals of Insight Groups are:

■ *To consider the sources of the drug problem*. This is not an essential goal that must be completed by the last Insight Group session, but the young person should have an opportunity to consider how fear, boredom or pain may have given rise to his or her involvement with chemicals. The Insight Group should provide an arena in which these issues can be raised, if not resolved.

■ *To uncover serious problems that may be related to drug use*. By the end of the Insight Group cycle, those involved should have some idea about whether or not physical or sexual abuse, suicidal thoughts, depression or other emotional problems are related to drug use. The counselor is not the expert in these areas and thus, is not responsible for assessing these problems, but the counselor should refer the young person for appropriate help. Such issues are best handled in private counseling sessions.

■ *To make decisions*. Not every problem can be resolved by the end of a group cycle. Of course, abstinence from drugs is expected of all participants during the group and afterward. Other specific actions, such as therapy, treatment or participation in a support group, vary with each young person. Making decisions about taking the next appropriate step after participation in an Insight Group is an important part of the process.

The development of *self*-awareness, then, is a major goal of the Insight Group process. Certainly, specific information about drug use can be obtained in brief, efficient interviews with the young person, with parents, with teachers, with friends and with brothers and sisters. However, the initial fear and anger that a young person feels when the drug issue is raised may block his or her comprehension of this information. The nine-session cycle of an Insight Group provides a means of breaking down barriers to awareness and of increasing the young person's ability to utilize the new information.

Intervention groups for the children of alcoholics

Intervention groups for the children of alcoholics are usually called concerned persons groups; they serve people concerned about another person's drinking and/or use of other drugs. Another type of group for young people who live with alcoholic parents is Alateen, which emphasizes the twelve steps of recovery advocated by the Al-Anon organization. (In most communities, the phone numbers of local Alateen, Al-Anon and Alcoholics Anonymous contacts are listed in the phone book.)

Reaching the children of alcoholics is an opportunity that we urge every school district and court service to take advantage of, no matter how great the pressures are to cut funding. Most of these young people will be neglected if early-intervention programs do not help them.

Problems with adult treatment centers

The treatment centers that help alcoholic adults have seldom offered significant assistance to their clients' children. As one school counselor explained, "Treating the parents' alcoholism certainly takes care of the more obvious problems of the parents, but it often does not have a strong impact on children's feelings. I remember working with a student who was the daughter of an alcoholic. Her father went in for treatment, but she continued to have the same kinds of feelings when her father was sober as she did when he was drinking. The changes that happened for her father did not happen for her."

According to the research report "Services for Children of Alcoholics" (National Institute on Alcohol Abuse and Alcoholism, 1981), some treatment centers still focus primarily on the alcoholic to the neglect of his or her children. The report also stated: "After considering a broad range of settings ..., schools and recreational programs generally were thought to be the most promising" for identifying children of alcoholic parents.

Isolation, embarrassment and resentment

Putting the children of alcoholics together in a group can have a powerful effect on them. The research report "An Assessment of the Needs of and Resources for Children of Alcoholic Parents" (Booz-Allen and Hamilton, 1974), cited "resentment and embarrassment" concerning their parents as the emotions most frequently expressed by a sample of 50 children of alcoholics. This embarrassment leads children to try to keep their family's problem a secret, which in turn increases their feelings of isolation. Also, the children of alcoholics are more likely than children of

nonalcoholics to become alcoholics themselves or to marry alcoholics (see data in Chapter Three).

Group Process

A concerned persons or Alateen group can be very frustrating and painful for a facilitator because of the difficulty of establishing a clear focus and finding some resolution. A person whose pain is related to another's drinking has little control over the situation and cannot expect quick and satisfying solutions. Group counselors must learn to avoid rushing in and smoothing things over for these young people, since awareness of pain is an important step toward growth and progress. Counselors, who must let people leave a session still carrying their pain, often find that a great deal of growth occurs between group sessions.

No matter what counseling style or group technique a facilitator uses, he or she should keep the following goals in mind when dealing with children of alcoholics:

- *Let them know that they are not alone*. Assure them that others share their experiences and understand their feelings.

- *Validate their experiences*. Listen to them, let them talk. Help them sort out their confusion and explain that, although they feel crazy, they are not. Rather, they are reacting to parents who downplay or ignore the severity of their own problems, deny that certain events ever took place and behave inconsistently.

- *Help them gain some perspective on how their parent's alcoholism has affected them*. It has often been said that children from alcoholic families fall into predictable, unhealthy patterns of behavior as a reaction to this problem. Some become overly responsible to compensate for the irresponsibility of a parent; others act out constantly to get attention from an otherwise inattentive parent. Groups for children of alcoholics can help participants identify these patterns and consider ways of changing their behavior.

- *Try to absolve them of blame*. Convince

them that their mother's or father's drinking is not their fault and that they cannot control it.

■ *Help them separate the parent from the drunken behavior*. Make it clear that their parent's drinking is not a sign that they are not loved by the parent. Ask them to remember, if they can, what it was like at home before their mother or father started drinking heavily.

■ *Offer them hope*. Let them know that alcoholism is a disease from which their parent can recover.

■ *Urge them to take care of themselves*. Encourage them to do positive things for themselves and stop any of their own behavior that enables their mother or father to continue drinking.

■ *Provide them with a safe outlet for dealing with their anger*. Help them deal with their anger at both the alcoholic parent and the nonalcoholic parent who has not protected them or made things better.

■ *Explain their own risks of becoming chemically dependent*. Make them aware that they are at high risk of becoming chemically dependent or of marrying a chemically dependent person. Older children of alcoholics who are about to leave home tend to believe that their troubles will soon be over. They need to know that they are more likely to encounter certain problems than children raised in families in which alcoholism is not present. This has to be handled very judiciously. Be careful not to use the label "child of an alcoholic" as though that particular aspect of their lives totally defines their present identity and future actions. Nonetheless, it must be made clear that, for a variety of reasons, the children of alcoholics are at higher risk than others of becoming chemically dependent.

■ *Build their self-esteem*. Help raise the self-esteem of these children in whatever way possible. Simply having an adult listen closely to them can boost the self-esteem of many of these children.

Referral and Coordination with Outside Agencies

After making a preliminary assessment and referring the young person and family to outside services, early-intervention programs could conceivably bow out of the ensuing action. However, outside agencies will need the background information gathered by early-intervention program staff members. The families will probably need some support and encouragement in making the crucial next step. The young person, when returning to the school or other referring system, will need some support in making changes and making them stick. And, to provide the youth with appropriate support, the early-intervention program staff will also need information from the outside agencies. Therefore, although program staff members could cease all assistance after a referral has been made, it benefits everyone if they coordinate referrals with outside agencies.

List of resources

When people face crises in their lives, they often use all of their emotional resources dealing with the stress and so find it very difficult to muster the energy or initiative needed to begin searching for help. To help people make this first step, schools, courts and social service agencies frequently provide booklets or information packets that describe local resources related to drug use and family problems, and explain how to contact them.

All of these available service agencies should be contacted in the initial phases of program organization, well before any young people are referred for services. It may fall to the program task force or the program coordinator to assess the strengths and weaknesses of each agency, the extent to which each is prepared to deal with adolescents and how agency staff members feel about working closely with a school or court program. To make appropriate and helpful referrals, the school or court must also know who is and who is not eligible for services and under what conditions; what fees are charged; and whether or not insurance policies cover the cost of services.

Once a suggestion for action is made, the early-intervention staff should follow it up to see if the young person or the family made contact, if the service suggested was appropriate and if the outside service needs further help from the referring counselor.

Sharing information

Schools, courts and social service agencies should establish procedures that allow them to share confidential information in a manner consistent with clients' needs and rights. As one program counselor told us, "Nothing will sabotage a program sooner than not being able to get information back and forth between people. Assessment counselors need to know what a young person's problems were in school and school people need to know how to integrate post-treatment plans into the school's schedule. This is a significant issue and counselors invest a lot of time maintaining a feeling of trust and cooperation with community agencies. Standard procedures for the release of confidential information forms should be established, and regular meetings with those agencies should be conducted."

When people begin making changes in their lives, they frequently need encouragement and support. Even if the early-intervention program is not providing any specific services, occasional brief contacts with staff members who offer a sympathetic ear can be a big boost to people who have been referred to agencies outside the school or courts.

Support Services

Whether a young person is returning to the community from a treatment program or from a juvenile detention center with a drug intervention program or has stopped using chemicals while remaining in school, she or

he needs some support.

A person who is returning from a treatment program needs a great deal of assistance in the first few weeks after treatment. Straightening out class schedules, getting credit for work done while in treatment and dealing with the shock of returning to a community and school where drugs are available all place tremendous pressure on the person, pressure that school staff members, probation officers and counselors can do much to alleviate.

For the young person who remains in school, meeting with a counselor for five or ten minutes several times a week can be very helpful. Little insight-oriented counseling is needed. Usually the knowledge that someone is aware of his or her efforts to remain drug-free and is willing to help if problems arise is sufficient.

Among the best services a school can offer to young people trying to remain drug-free is a student support group for drug-free living. These can be either aftercare groups for young people out of treatment or abstinence support groups for others. Students who have never used chemicals can benefit from "Still Straight Groups," as can young people who appear at risk for drug use. Young people manifesting one or more risk factors (see Chapter Three) should be encouraged to participate.

Support groups for drug-free living

Some of the possible needs that a student support group can meet are:

▪ *A new peer group*. A support group can offer a young person who wishes to stay away from chemicals the opportunity to meet others of similar bent. Together they can establish a new drug-free peer group.

▪ *Focus on personal goals*. The group can supply support, encouragement and a real push to help each member work on such goals as improving attendance at school or cooperation at home; exploring new activities or helping promote new activities to enjoy while remaining drug-free; or finding a regular or youth-oriented AA group that feels comfortable.

■ *Confrontation*. Group members can confront one another about any behaviors that may lead to a relapse of drug use.

■ *Monitoring*. A regularly scheduled group provides an ongoing and convenient way of checking in with students. The participants' personal knowledge of one another and their connection with the peer grapevine can be useful in keeping tabs on behavior related to drug use and other issues.

■ *Emotional contact*. Support groups are a milieu in which personal, feeling-oriented communication and personal connections can be developed. One of the most common disappointments of young people returning from treatment is that it is not considered normal in the "outside world" to talk about feelings, to hug others or to share the intimate details of one's life. The process of sharing can be more important than the content shared.

Group composition

Conceivably, a variety of young people can participate in an abstinence support group: chemically dependent kids who have been through treatment; those who are not clearly chemically dependent but have had some drug problems that they are concerned about; high-risk students who have an alcoholic parent or, for some other reason, wish to maintain a drug-free lifestyle and feel they need the support even though they have not yet used drugs; students who simply want to join a clique and get a peer group; students who come directly from an Insight Group or from an AA group in the community. Those who are staying straight without treatment may work well together, while those who have been to treatment may benefit from having a group of their own. Students who have been in treatment share a vocabulary and an intense experience that other students may find alien, at least at first.

Daily activities

A look at the needs a support group can meet in a young person's life suggests agenda items for daily group activities. Often, the concerns that young people bring to their group carry the meeting on most days. There are enough issues concerning drugs in the schools to keep groups busy for a long time. One of the dangers in a support group, however, is that the group may turn to a one-to-one format in which the facilitator and the young person who raises an issue interact, excluding other group members. To avoid the one-to-one format, facilitators can regularly use a variety of techniques to help include all group members in the process.

When beginning a support group for the week, even before the group starts to deal with a group member who has a pressing need, the facilitator may find it helpful to conduct a brief "survey" of how members fared during the week. Some ideas for this procedure are:

○ Have each person share "high" and "low" points since the last meeting.

○ Ask each group member to share one significant thing that happened during the week.

○ Suggest that group members share a new discovery about themselves that they made during the week.

○ Have participants describe the new risks they took during the week.

○ Have each group member say how he or she is feeling on a scale from 1 to 10.

A similar procedure can be used to close a group meeting. At the end of a session, the facilitator can ask each group member to take one new risk during the week and relate the experience at the beginning of the next session. Participants can also be asked to try to make one new discovery about themselves during the week.

In dealing with a specific group member, the facilitator can ask other group members to give some feedback. To ensure that all members are participating, some facilitators suggest that, starting on the right, they go around the group and have each member give some feedback to the young person in question. In such an exercise, it is also useful for the person receiving the feedback to remain silent until the group has finished. Sometimes this can be structured so that the feedback solicited is positive feedback only.

In closing the group, a request for process statements is also useful. By process statements, we mean comments on how the group went about its business rather than on what was discussed. For instance, if the group addressed some very painful material, it still may be appropriate to ask, "How did we do today?" The group may have worked very well and it may have been a "good" group session, even if the material did not leave everyone feeling happy. How the students define a "good" session provides insights as to how the group process is working: Did everyone participate? Did people who gave feedback take new risks? Is the group being honest? Is the group focused on maintaining a drug-free lifestyle? Do people feel safe in the group? These are the kinds of issues that must concern facilitators and they are also the kinds of issues that are best answered when the whole group participates.

Special group days

As the weeks go by in support groups, a backlog of unfinished business sometimes builds up and, because the sessions are limited to one hour or less, there is little opportunity to catch up. Occasionally, perhaps once per quarter or semester, facilitators schedule a "field trip" for all members in the group. Members obtain permission to be absent from their classes for the day and go to some outside location for a daylong group. Much unfinished business can be taken care of and considerable growth can occur under these circumstances.

Special activities

Groups can undertake activities other than their own group agendas. They can have their own drug-free parties; plan prevention programs for the school; go on picnics or other outings; and work with community groups on drug problems.

Referral to community agencies

Support groups focusing primarily on maintaining a drug-free lifestyle have very full agendas. When deep emotional or family issues arise, it is seldom appropriate for the group to address them in detail. Although many of these important issues are considered in treatment, it is very likely that they will surface again in a support group. Although group members can offer some feedback and support, the group cannot do a great deal about resolving such problems. Sometimes in this situation a referral to professionals in the community is warranted.

Sometimes a facilitator has an intuition that a particular student has a serious personal or family problem. If so, one or both facilitators, if there is a co-facilitator, should talk to the student privately and consider referral to an outside agency. If the issue is one for which strict state guidelines have been established—such as the need for immediate referral in cases of child abuse—laws may dictate what action must be taken. However, other issues will involve voluntary action on the part of the student or the parents. It is helpful if the facilitator or someone else in the school has rapport with a local mental health or social service agency so that such referrals can be handled smoothly.

Self-help groups

Involvement in young people's AA, Al-Anon and many other self-help groups can contribute to staying drug free. However, a young person should be given some guidance and support when attempting to utilize local self-help groups. Although most of these groups have a general philosophy supported by literature distributed by some central organization, local groups have a great deal of flexibility as to how they define their membership and goals. Some adults who have been in a self-help group for years are not very warm and accepting of young people whose drinking and drug use history differs considerably from that of the adults in the group. Some AA groups want to deal only with problems related to alcohol, while others are open to discussions about drugs other than alcohol. Some groups are very personally and emotionally stressful, while others eschew personal interaction and focus on discussions of a twelve-step philosophy.

Young people need advice from a counselor and/or parents when trying to determine whether it would be helpful to join a new self-help group. Members of various groups often have strong ideas about what has been good for them as individuals and as a group, and they may insist that young newcomers accept these ideas. Discussion with an adult outside the group gives a young person a chance to reflect on and respond to the implicit assumptions of the group.

Other types of groups

Insight Groups, concerned persons groups and abstinence support groups are the mainstays of the early-intervention approach. Early-intervention programs have, however, set up a variety of other group models when the need arose. These groups include "Families in Change" groups, for young people whose families are undergoing a divorce or separation; self-esteem groups; and school adjustment groups, for students who have recently moved into a school district. No particular group model must be considered permanent unless the need for it is constant. It makes sense to start groups, continue them until interest or need lags, and then discontinue them.

General Comments on Groups

The role of facilitators

Facilitators give structure and direction to groups. They do more than merely facilitate, they also teach and lead. The technique of letting people struggle to select a leader is not appropriate here. The facilitator should explicitly describe the goals of the group and the hoped-for process; provide agendas and norms for group interaction; and help the group stay focused on those agendas. Peer interaction is crucial, but the adult facilitator is an important member of the group. No matter how rebellious the participants appear, they will respect an adult facilitator. His or her opinions and information will carry significant weight. To make use of this position, facilitators should have some capacity for confrontation as well as for accurate empathy.

One common way to facilitate support groups is to have a trained school staff member work with a drug treatment professional from the community. This practice has several advantages: The facilitators teach each other about their respective milieus (the school environment and the treatment environment), and the different perspectives they offer are helpful to group members.

Professionals from treatment centers often volunteer so that they can maintain contact with the schools and gain insights into what services they should be offering to young people.

Age and number of participants

The minimum age requirement for groups depends on the purpose of the group. There are groups for the very young children of alcoholics—those in third, fourth or fifth grades—but they take on a different tone than the groups we have described here. For the most part, groups that require the ability to express feelings, to comment on group processes and to engage in some type of confrontation are appropriate for students 12 or 13 years of age or older.

Also, it is usually appropriate to separate junior high school students from senior high school students.

Groups may sometimes form out of the personal preferences of the participants, such as when a group wishes to remain for girls only or when a group of friends want to stay

together. There is no reason to deny these
personal preferences if the group works well
and its exclusivity is not perceived by others
as a clique. Therapy groups, of course, are an
entirely different case, but when the goal is
simply to support drug-free living, a certain
measure of self-determination should be respected.

Groups with only two or three people are
too small to generate sufficient group action.
Six to ten people per group is probably opti-
mum, while 12 approaches the upper limit.
Larger groups should be divided into smaller
groups.

Scheduling and other issues

Quite often, support groups are given a low
priority in a student's schedule. They must be
squeezed in before classes begin, during the
lunch hour or after the school day is completed. Such scheduling patterns are very un-
desirable and discourage success. Support
groups are best scheduled during the school
day.

A common time to schedule groups is mid-
morning on Wednesday. The first period of
the day can pose problems because lively interaction early in the morning comes hard to
many people. The second, third and fourth
periods of the morning seem to work the best.

There are a variety of ways to handle the
details of scheduling these classes:

■ *Rotating schedule*. Groups may not have a
fixed time every week, because the teachers
whose students are absent from their classes
during that time may object. For this reason
the support groups may "flow" throughout
the schedule. Students miss one class one
week and another the next. This can be difficult to implement, however, if it causes

teachers involved with the groups to miss the
classes they usually teach.

■ *Passes*. In some schools, students receive a
pass ahead of time from the early-intervention program coordinator. They report to
their class, hand the pass to the teacher and
then leave class to go to their group. In other
schools, teachers simply mark off who is absent. Absence lists are checked against the attendance sheets for support groups.

■ *Frequency*. Most support groups take place
weekly, which, during some stages of problem resolution, is not sufficient. Sometimes a
student needs support *every day*, such as
when returning from a treatment program.
For this reason, sometimes an informal half-
hour meeting is held in the program facilitator's or other core team member's office before the class day begins.

■ *Offering credit*. Some schools offer credit
to students participating in support groups
because the interpersonal, health and social
issues raised there are considered to be a significant contribution to the general educational process.

* * *   * * *   * * *

No matter how diverse the services offered by
an early-intervention program, how high the
quality of those services and how good the
relationship between the early-intervention
staff members and local service providers,
much of the impact of the program is nulli-
fied if parents are not involved. In the next
chapter we look at the issue of parental involvement in the early-intervention process.
We also describe how parents can participate
in mobilizing a community to be more effective in addressing drug problems.

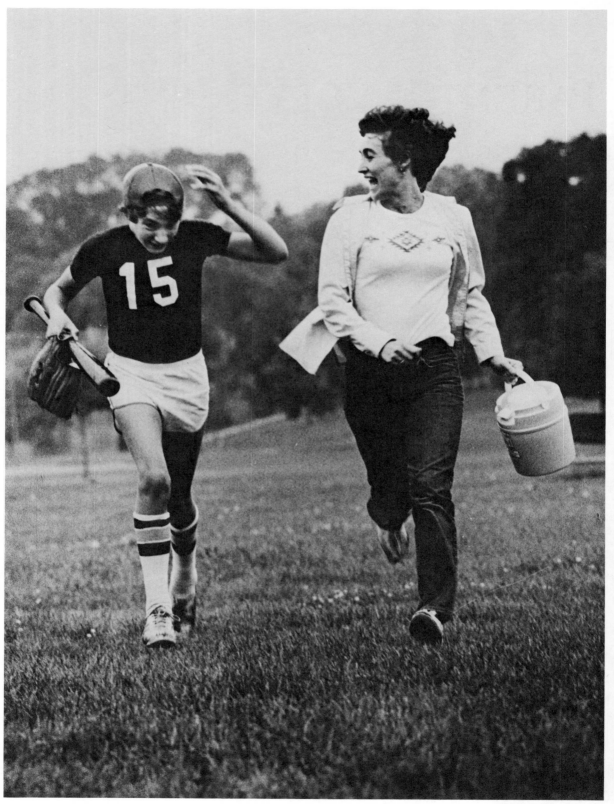

photo: Jeffrey Grosscup

CHAPTER EIGHT

PARENT INVOLVEMENT
A Key to Success

Two things are becoming clear as early-intervention programs develop: First, parent cooperation is necessary to do anything to help a particular drug-using student. Second, parent support is essential in making significant changes in the community and is often the single driving force behind those changes.

"Once the parents got involved, we began to get some action." This quote is typical of many we have heard from people across the country. Parents can be our number one allies in working with young people and in developing early-intervention programs. Often, when administrative backup is lacking, parents' support for programs convinces administrators to stand behind front-line counselors. However, before parents understand the issues of chemical use and the nature of early intervention, they can be confused about, threatened by and hostile toward intervention into their own children's drug problems. Therefore, it is important to involve parents at the beginning of and throughout the process of program development.

In this chapter we deal with three major aspects of parent involvement: working with parents whose children are or may be using drugs; working with students whose parents may have a drinking problem; and working with parents groups that focus on community action.

Attitudinal Barriers

When the fear of teachers and other staff members is combined with the defensiveness and guilt of parents, formidable barriers arise that make it difficult to involve parents in the early-intervention process.

Teachers who become afraid of parents

Certainly, a teacher who fails to act on an obvious drug abuse problem or who intentionally avoids areas in the school where drug use is known to occur may be lazy and uninvolved, a drug or alcohol abuser or simply reluctant to confront people. It is more likely, however, that this teacher has already confronted young people about drugs, with one of four results:

○ The parents became extremely angry and manipulated the administration into agreeing that the teacher was out of line and should not have been concerned about the student's drug use.

○ The teacher finally believes fellow teachers who time and again have said that so many students are doing drugs that it is a waste of time to work with any single problem that arises.

○ The teacher has reported students for drug use and they were expelled immediately without being offered help.

○ The teacher has referred drug users to an overworked, overwrought or jaded assistant principal who did nothing more than send them back to the classroom.

Teachers can become very frightened of parents if they do not know how the parents will react and if they do not know whether the administration will back them up. Clear, fair, consistently applied policies are essential in working with the parents of teenage drug abusers. Parent involvement from the beginning of program development is advisable. It is also helpful if school drug policies are made available to parents *before* their children get into trouble. A letter sent out every year, to remind parents of the presence of drug abuse policies and appropriate services, can be a great facilitator of intervention as the school year progresses. General or special sessions for parents, such as meetings involving coaches and the parents of athletes, can produce a more cooperative environment for working with drug users and their parents.

The feelings of parents of drug abusers

When young people are cited for a violation of the laws or regulations concerning the use of alcohol and other drugs, their parents face a twofold crisis: a crisis within the family and a crisis between the family and the outside world. Within the family, parents have concerns about their own responsibility for the drug problems, fears that other children in the family may become "contaminated" by the drug use of a sibling and confusion over what to do about the drug user. In the outside world, they feel they are being criticized or

ridiculed and they worry about how the decisions of the schools and the courts will affect their lives. Their external behavior often indicates:

■ *denial*—the parents deny that any problem exists;

■ *shock*—parents are totally surprised and have little comment; or

■ *blaming*—they are immediately angry and blame someone else for the problem.

Underlying all these reactions is pain. Parents of drug users who have been caught feel awkward and ashamed. These negative feelings can lead to hostile reactions at first. Their response is to be expected and is not a sign that they do not love their children and are not good parents. It is also not a clear prognosticator; many parents who are originally hostile to the interveners eventually become staunch program supporters.

Professionals who attempt to intervene with adolescent drug abusers must take into account the effects of their actions, not only on the young person but also on the parents. When working with adolescents, some of us tend naturally to assume the role of youth advocate: advocacy of legal rights and the right of self-determination or general advocacy for young people against any negative pressures impinging on them. At first blush, advocacy seems to be an unassailably positive stance. However, it can easily slide into advocacy *for* the youth *against* the parents. If this happens, counselors and educators can lose sight of the need to support both the parents and their children when intervening for drug problems.

One type of parental reaction, perhaps the one that poses the most problems, is detachment or unconcern. When parents show little concern about their child's drug use, getting them involved in intervention is likely to be difficult. Despite the tendency to become defensive, some parents have a very positive, hopeful reaction when contacted about their child. These parents express genuine concern about their child having used alcohol or other drugs and evince a mature assessment of the situation. Some parents say that they have become increasingly worried and have tried, without success, to clamp down on their child's behavior. Others admit to being concerned, and while they do not believe that their child is dependent or a chronic user, they are willing to have the school continue with its evaluation.

People working in early-intervention programs do not have to assess family dynamics, offer therapy to the family or solve the parents' problems. Yet they cannot be totally oblivious to the possible effects of their actions on families. In the next section we discuss how an early-intervention program staff can involve the parents of drug users in the intervention process.

Parents in the Intervention Process

No matter how good your policy development has been and how conscientious you have been in trying to enlist parent support for the program, the first contact with parents concerning drug use or possible drug use can be very intimidating to both the school staff member and the parents. Such contacts commonly take place when:

o a student has been caught while intoxicated or using drugs on the school grounds;

o a student has shown a marked decline in academic performance or a disinterest in other activities and there seems to be some disruptive personal problems; or

o a student has admitted to being concerned about his or her drug use.

The way in which a student's drug problem comes to light has a significant impact on how school personnel contact the parents and bring them into the intervention process. The reasons for contacting the parents also vary and further affect the nature of the contact. The following five general reasons for contacting the parents may be useful for guiding the nature of specific contacts:

■ *The parents' right to know*. Common sense and explicit laws usually require that the parents be notified immediately when their child has violated the law and/or is experiencing significant health problems. While this is always the case when a student is caught using drugs or intoxicated, it may or may not be true in cases of self-referral or performance decline.

■ *Assessment-intervention considerations*. Parents can contribute greatly to the assessment-intervention process. They have data and the school has data; the whole is greater than the sum of its parts. When a staff member contacts parents, he or she should give them some guidelines for accumulating more information about their child's recent behavior.

■ *To clarify parental responsibilities*. Parents must be made aware of their responsibilities and prerogatives in regard to controlling and helping to change their child's behavior.

■ *To clarify the school's responsibilities and prerogatives*. Parents must be made aware of what actions the school can and will take given their cooperation or noncooperation.

■ *To enlist parent support*. It is extremely advantageous if the parents become willing participants in the assessment-intervention process and if their cooperation begins with the very first phone call.

Child caught using or intoxicated

When a student is found to be intoxicated or in possession of drugs on the school grounds, many schools require that the parents come immediately and take the child out of school. In this situation, school personnel have time to inform the parents about the incident and explain the general process that will follow; in-depth discussions of the nature of the child's drug use problem must wait. There may also be some issues regarding police involvement that must be addressed. In any event, this is not the time to conduct even the briefest screening interview. The distinguishing characteristic of this situation is that the immediate concern is clear: The student has violated a school policy and probably a state or federal law.

Whoever is making the first contact with the parents should already know the exact details of the situation and be able to let the parents know what will follow if the parents cooperate or if they do not. Ambiguity in this situation can be very intimidating. Three simple points to be communicated are:

○ Since the student was apprehended while intoxicated or in possession of drugs, a problem exists and the school must take action immediately.

○ Although the facts of the immediate incident are incontrovertible, the full extent of the problem is not known at this time.

○ Certain standard procedures must be followed.

In any event, at the first contact it is good to let parents know the procedures and the reasons for the meeting or meetings being scheduled. It is not likely that a great deal of work can be done at the very first phone call because the parents may be in a state of shock. The parents' reaction to the initial contact may determine whether or not the school can immediately move into a cooperative assessment effort or will have to keep the interaction based on contractual, legalistic terms requiring minimum involvement on the part of the parents.

If the contact person fears the parents' anger or believes that they will appeal successfully to a higher authority in the school system, the chances are greater that she or he will attempt to intimidate them in some manner. The contact person should keep the following in mind: *In general, do not let the overzealous use of legitimate power block the likelihood of willing cooperation.*

Performance or behavioral problems

When a student shows a degeneration in academic performance or behavior, the schools have good reason for requesting parent cooperation. In the process of early intervention, we want to try to help students *before* they drop below the minimum requirements. We want to offer assistance when a student stops performing up to his or her potential or when there is a marked decline from previous performance levels. With such general criteria as a decline in academic performance, it is possible that current problems are related to issues having nothing to do with drugs. Therefore, the decision to refer for assessment of drug-related problems must be deferred until other possibilities have been considered.

The three main criteria for performance referrals in early-intervention programs are: an increase in absences, a decline in grades and an increase in disciplinary problems. If the school has some mechanism for warning parents about their child's behavior in regard to these areas, parents have an opportunity to intervene before the school has to take further action. It is helpful if the initial contacts do not come from a centralized source, such as a school administrator, but rather from individual teachers or coaches. When parents hear the information from a variety of sources, they cannot fault any one person. When problems start to arise, then, parents can be given *opportunities* to discuss them with teachers before the administration demands that parents appear for discussions.

Self-referrals

When students ask for help with alcohol or drug problems, they often expect the kind of help they *want* rather than the kind of help they *need*. How and when the parents should be brought into the intervention process is not always a simple issue. Certainly, if the student is clearly a danger to herself or himself or to others, parents must be notified immediately. If it seems advisable that the student join one of the formal support groups in the school, such as an Insight Group, it is often necessary to obtain the parents' permission.

Some young people are concerned about their own drug use but there are no indications that they have ever driven while under the influence of a drug or that their grades are being markedly affected. Some professionals maintain that parent notification should be automatic and immediate even in these cases, because it is the parents' right to know. Others interpret federal or state confidentiality guidelines to mean that the school can never reveal such information to the parents. Whatever your district's position and whatever your personal viewpoint, keep in mind the two dangers lurking at the opposite ends of this issue:

○ If you do not believe in notifying or bringing parents into the intervention process simply because you believe it is the young person's issue to deal with, there is a great likelihood that you will be helping the student maintain the *status quo* by helping him or her feel better on occasion.

○ If you believe, on principle alone, that parents should be notified automatically and immediately, students may hesitate to admit to having problems with drugs. If the policy allows no discretion and students know that parent involvement is inevitable and immediate, the staff's ability to help students who do not manifest the more obvious behavioral problems related to drugs and alcohol is severely limited. If students have some opportunity to work with a counselor or a support group to prepare themselves for telling their parents about serious issues, the parent-child interaction is less likely to degenerate into the established patterns of argument, denial or other negative responses. Parents can be drawn into the process in a constructive rather than a destructive manner.

Some counselors prefer to notify parents whenever a student has a drug problem. However, instead of contacting the parents directly, they urge the student to tell the parents, and they support the student in doing so. When a student is not in a situation that mandates the parents being notified but has admitted concern about drug use, the counselor can say: "I think you should tell your parents about this. Why don't you do it during the next 24 hours and come back and see me tomorrow. I want you to think about it." Another technique is for the counselor to call the parents while the student is present. The counselor is then perceived as an intermediary who takes the load off the student rather than as a snitch.

First meeting with parents

When a drug violation is involved, a meeting is usually set up several days, or even a week, after the initial contact. At that time the situation is discussed in depth. A person with clear administrative authority should be present and probably should conduct the meeting. This lets the parents know that they are already near or at the top of the ladder in terms of appeals and that the school considers it an important issue. When a drug violation or other disciplinary issue is not involved, the first meeting with the parents can be structured in a variety of ways, often with a counselor alone or with a counselor and concerned staff member, such as a coach or a teacher.

It is probably best to schedule the meeting after the in-school data-gathering process has been completed. This information should be available to the parents during the meeting so that they can participate more fully in the decision-making process. Some schools suspend the student until that time, but this policy creates some problems. Such suspensions often put a tremendous burden on the parents while the student is allowed to roam free.

The first in-depth meeting with parents includes a report on the data collected, a report of the face-to-face interview with the student and, sometimes, the student's own interpretation of events. It is extremely important that *both* parents attend this session. Even if separated or divorced, both parents may still be involved in parenting and thus should be at the initial conference. If not, the one parent may never even tell the other about the incident or the information may not be relayed to the other parent without being altered considerably. If this happens, the parent who was not present and consequently cannot fully understand the situation may not cooperate with efforts to intervene into the young person's drug problems. It is quite common for parents to offer excuses as to why only one of them can attend: The husband is out of town. The wife cannot possibly take time off from her job. Such excuses should be challenged and specific details requested: When will he be back? Can we reach him by a long-distance phone call? Can you take sick time from your job to come to this conference?

Part of the early-intervention process is to ensure that all of the normal and potentially helpful procedures have been tried with a student before a general conference is called. If contact with the parents becomes necessary when the data are not as clear as in cases in which the student has violated a school rule, the contact takes on a different tone; the early-intervention program staff members and school authorities must be more flexible in what they expect from the parents and the child. Nonetheless, if the staff is convinced that the information points to a serious health problem, then the school still has its prerogatives and should take a firm stand.

After the conference with the parents, staff participants can support one another by talking about feelings; sharing praise and encouragement; and giving constructive feedback. Do a follow-up with the student. Do not expect a quick fix.

When there is an ongoing behavioral or academic problem and neither the student nor the parents can see or admit to a serious health, emotional or drug problem, a series of conferences may be necessary.

Involving parents in the assessment process

If cooperative, parents can be very helpful in the assessment process. Parents can be asked for data that may indicate a drug or other personal problem in their child's life: Have they been missing money? Has their liquor been disappearing mysteriously? Has their child found new friends who are considerably different from old friends, and have they ever been introduced to them? Are there many telephone calls from a lot of different kids whom the parents do not know? Have calls been coming at all hours of the day and night? Have there been many more problems with curfew and with general cooperation around the house? Do siblings, younger and older, have any perceptions they can share?

Parent cooperation must also be enlisted to ensure that the young person follows through on suggestions for assistance. If a student is to attend an Insight Group for three weeks, parents should be supportive of the suggestion. If a young person is to avoid a particular drug hangout, parents should enforce that requirement. If it is recommended that the young person and the family seek counseling, parents should follow through on arranging for counseling. Sometimes it is helpful to list the areas where parent cooperation is requested or required so that the parents have a clear idea of what is expected of them.

Interventions for Parents' Alcohol Problems

One problem that consistently frustrates those working in school-based early-intervention programs is the difficulty of intervening with parents whose drinking is having a negative effect on their children. Many educators feel that confronting parents with concrete data about their children's drug problems is risky enough; confronting parental alcoholism is akin to stepping into a political minefield.

The director of a social service agency explained how services outside the school can be helpful in such situations: "There's no question that community agencies have an advantage over the schools when it comes to working with problem-drinking or alcoholic parents. Even when it seems obvious that parental alcoholism is affecting a student's school behavior, it is not always easy to get parents to see the relationship between drinking and their children's behavior and to see why school personnel should be concerned at all.

"Schools can begin an intervention, however, by referring the young person to us on the basis of a manifested behavioral problem. Kids with school avoidance problems, for instance, have been sent to us for counseling when there was suspicion that the parents' drinking was the heart of the problem.

"We can be very effective when kids come here for their own problems first rather than for the issue of parental alcoholism. Once we start working with them, we can call their parents and say, 'There are some issues we're working on with your kid and we need your help to go further.' They come in here because of the difficulties that their children are having and those are legitimate problems that need to be addressed. It is also very legitimate for us to relate their drinking to their kids' problems whenever appropriate."

Some school and court staff members decline to work with children of alcoholics because they feel they *must* intervene with the parents if they are to do any good at all. Since they do not want to get involved with the parents' personal lives, they just avoid the whole problem. This is very unfortunate. Simply by offering basic support services to these children, the schools and other community resources can be extremely helpful regardless of the parents' problems. The point is, do not do nothing because you think you have to do everything once you get involved.

Parents Groups

Over the past 10 to 15 years, a variety of groups have been organized to help parents with such problems as the learning disabili-

ties or incurable diseases of their children. Alcohol and drug problems among adolescents have also given rise to a number of parents groups whose focuses range from mutual support for dealing with a drug-using adolescent to nationwide political action. Most parents groups emphasize one of the following functions:

- *Mutual support.* Some parents groups are formed by the families of adolescent drug abusers to give mutual support and guidance.
- *Establishment of clear norms for adolescents.* Some parents groups are formed by parents, who may or may not have a child who is a drug abuser, to help establish clear community norms regarding adolescent behavior and to help support early-intervention activities in schools and elsewhere.
- *Information and education.* Many parents groups focus on educating themselves and others about drugs and drug problems.
- *Political action.* Some groups are formed to effect broad political changes. They are active in such areas as regulating the sale of drug paraphernalia; influencing and strengthening legislative and police efforts at drug control; fighting the problem of drunk driving; and creating laws and regulations concerning the dissemination of information on drug abuse.

Support groups for parents

Parents whose children are involved with drugs can receive a great deal of help from one another. Support groups for parents help break through the isolation, shame and guilt of their families by offering feedback and helpful confrontation.

Families Anonymous is a national network of self-help groups serving parents and other close relatives of youths with drug problems and problems associated with drug use, such as rebelliousness and running away. A major technique of Families Anonymous groups is the use of the "twelve-steps," similar to those of Alcoholics Anonymous. The steps help alleviate the guilt, despair, anxiety and frustration common among spouses, parents, siblings and others close to drug abusers. Family members are encouraged to reduce their overprotective behavior and their sense of being responsible for drug-using individuals.

There are no statistics on the subject, but it appears that increasing numbers of parents whose kids are experiencing problems with drugs are either joining a Families Anonymous group in their area or starting one of their own. Although a national organization does publish literature for Families Anonymous groups, some groups are not formally affiliated with the national organization. These unaffiliated groups tend to develop their own operating norms. For instance, instead of using a twelve-step format, a group in one community has developed its own methods of offering support, insight and information to parents seeking help. The weekly three-hour meetings of this group always involve some sharing of problems or accomplishments related to parenting or other issues. Outside resource people, such as social service professionals and educators, are also invited to share their insights with the group.

A major, ongoing struggle for parents is dealing with the concept of "detachment" in regard to their children's problems with drugs. Parents struggle constantly to shed feelings of guilt and responsibility for their children's problems, while taking responsibility for their roles as parents in resolving these problems. This is where Families Anonymous differs from Al-Anon, according to Jerry W., one of the founding members of the Rochester, Minnesota, Families Anonymous group:

"Detachment really is a different issue for parents than it is for spouses. This crucial point is probably the single item that separates the Families Anonymous groups from most Al-Anon groups. Most of us were going to Al-Anon groups and we kept hearing about the need to take care of ourselves and to forget about the person who was using drugs. We heard that we couldn't do anything about a spouse's drinking and if we chose to live with that person we had to take care of our-

selves. We have a different degree of responsibility with a child than we do with a spouse. Adolescents are still growing and maturing and we still have responsibility for influencing their lives. We can't really influence an adult's life in the same way we can our children's."

Like professionals who work with parents of drug abusers, Jerry emphasized parents' tremendous need to overcome feelings of isolation: "There is no question in my mind that part of being human is to feel, in some way, inadequate. When we experience certain situations, such as drug problems with our kids, we think we're the only ones who have the problem, the only ones who feel inadequate, the only ones with low self-esteem. Both by sharing concerns and by listening to others, parents find out very quickly that many others have the same feelings and have had the same experiences."

Prevention: changing community norms

Confusion is rife among parents. They are besieged by a myriad of books about parenting and by conflicting claims about the harmfulness of drugs. Their children confuse them further by telling them that "everybody else's parents" let them do this or that.

To eliminate this confusion, many parents are banding together in "parent peer groups" to determine norms for adolescent behavior in general and adolescent drug use in particular. Some parents have begun by finding out with whom their children associate and then contacting those parents to discuss issues of parenting and drug use. Curfews and rules against going to unchaperoned parties or parties where liquor is served are high on the discussion lists of most of these groups. From a sociological perspective, these parents groups are trying to change the norms in their immediate community and society in general.

Political action

Some parents groups, such as Families In Action, do not focus on the behavior and emotions of family members and users; rather, they emphasize community action for the prevention and eradication of drug abuse. The Families In Action philosophy encompasses the need to educate parents, children and others about the rising use of drugs by youngsters; about the commercial and social pressures that encourage such behavior; and about the social, psychological and physiological consequences of drug use. The general goals of this organization are to stop drug use among children and teenagers; counteract the pressures in society that condone and promote drug use; and create a drug-free environment in the home, school and community to encourage the healthy growth of children (Rusche, 1979).

Professional involvement in parent groups

Professionals in the schools, courts or treatment centers do not have to wait for a parents group to form in their area. Although the nature of parents groups usually requires that they be directed by the parents rather than by social service or school professionals, professionals usually have harmonious relationships with such groups. They are able to stimulate initial interest in the group, bring parents together to begin the groups, provide suggestions for the initial meetings and refer new members once the group is established. Professionals also can serve as consultants by providing special education sessions to help the group work through specific problems.

***   ***   ***

So far we have considered the basic concepts and components of early-intervention programming. In the next chapter we take a look at one school's intervention program to see how these concepts and components work in real life.

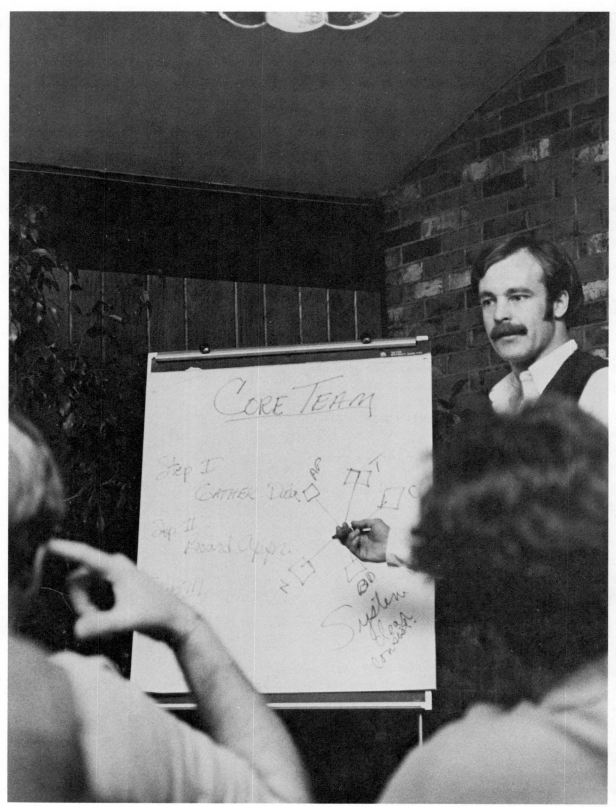

photo: Joseph Muldoon

CHAPTER NINE

PROGRAM ANALYSIS
One School District's Efforts

In this chapter we look at program evaluation data from the Minneapolis Public Schools' Chemical Awareness Program. Not only is the Minneapolis program one of the largest and most fully implemented early-intervention programs in the country, but it also has been using computers to store and analyze its information for the last four years.

Our analysis is descriptive rather than prescriptive. We do not attempt to prove that the Minneapolis school district is representative of other urban, suburban or rural districts around the country or that its program practices will have the same effects in other districts. Rather than attempting to analyze the Minneapolis program per se, we assess key issues and use the Minneapolis data for illustration.

Our purpose is to show how the early-intervention process works in practice; how people in the field begin by working with a large population of young people who may have disruptive personal problems, assess those problems and move the youths along to a wide range of different resources. We do this both by looking at profiles of the data collected by the Minneapolis program and by providing specific case examples.

The Minneapolis Program

In the 1983-84 school year, the Minneapolis Public Schools had an enrollment of 19,897 primary school students and 17,442 secondary school students in 62 different buildings. The early-intervention program staff has ranged from 16 to 24 people over the years, depending on budget allotments. During the 1983-84 school year, there were ten full-time counselors in the secondary schools and three counselors, some of whom worked only part-time, in the elementary schools. There were also three program support staff members. Note that these numbers do not, of course, include the many other school staff members and volunteers from the community who donated their time to the program. Nonetheless, it is clear that there is not a great amount of emphasis being placed on intervention in the elementary schools and the statistics given in this chapter may well have been different had more resources been allocated for younger children.

Program personnel perform identification and pre-assessment services and help facilitate chemical awareness groups (similar to the Insight Groups described in Chapter Seven), Alateen groups, concerned persons groups and abstinence support groups. They also present a wide range of inservice training for the public school staff, as well as awareness and education programs for parents and students.

Statistical Overview

A review of program statistics provides insights into the nature of this program. Additional commentary offers suggestions as to what these findings imply for the early-intervention process in general.

Number of clients

In the 1983-84 school year, the Minneapolis program served 1,919 clients. This figure includes about 200 students who were served at least twice during the year. The estimated number of elementary students seen one or more times was 296 or 1.5% of the elementary school population. The approximate number of secondary students served one or more times was 1,426, or 8% of the secondary student population. When the figures from all 12 grades are averaged, 4.6% of the entire student body received some service.

Approximately 5,000 students were reached through classroom presentations, health fairs and other educational activities. These activities probably contributed to the fairly high level of self-referrals described below.

Comments

This rate of intervention is sufficiently high. Students spend up to six years in secondary education. Even taking into account the fact that some portion of the 8% of students served annually in the secondary school program will be served again in another year during their time in the Minneapolis schools, no less than 8%—perhaps as many as 20% to 30% of a given class—are likely to undergo some form of screening for drug or other disruptive personal problems. As demonstrated later, this does *not* mean that such a large

proportion of students is being sent to treatment. It simply means that the possibility of their having disruptive personal problems is being addressed and clarified.

In addition to the students formally referred to the program, there are hundreds of other requests for consultations on the part of teachers and school administrators concerning the problems they face with students who may be having drug problems or other personal difficulties. Some of these "early-early" interventions will be very helpful to students and staff but will never be recorded in the statistics of the program. Nonetheless, this type of daily consultation is a significant contribution to the early-intervention process.

Age of clients

The average age of students served by the Minneapolis program in the 1983-84 school year was 13.9 years. The breakdown of average age by grade level was as follows: elementary, 9.4 years; junior high, 13.2 years; and senior high, 15.8 years. The combined average age of the junior and senior high students in the program was 14.8 years. In contrast, Kite (1980) found the average age of 250 adolescents in four different adolescent treatment centers, all of whom were at the secondary level, to be 16.3 years. It appears, then, that the Minneapolis Public Schools have a right to claim that they truly have an *early*-intervention program. Even though they, too, work with a population of drug users or those at high risk for drug use, their clients, on the average, are still one and one-half years younger than treatment program youth.

Comments

The students in the early-intervention program are neither identical to those in treatment programs nor representative of the student population as a whole. Analysis of the "age of first use" for the school program clients indicates that 87.2% of the students referred for their own drug use problems had used alcohol or other drugs by the end of eighth grade. This is considerably higher than comparable statistics from a nationwide study showing that 18.3% of the general student population had tried marijuana and 31.4% had tried alcohol by the end of eighth grade (Johnston, O'Malley and Bachman, 1984).

Sources of referrals

Most of the referrals to the Minneapolis program came from school staff members, of course, but a surprisingly large number came from other sources. The breakdown follows:

○ school staff, 62%;

○ voluntary: self, 15%; family, 12%; friends, 5%;

○ community agencies, 6%.

Elementary students had the highest percentage of family referrals (23%) compared with 10% each for junior and senior high students. Senior high students had the highest percentage of self-referrals (19%) compared with 12% for junior high and 9% for elementary students.

The source of referrals varies to some extent according to the major problem area of the students. Eleven percent of those with problems related to their own chemical use were self-referrals, while 19% of those concerned about another's drug use were self-referrals. Of those who had problems both with their own and with another's use of chemicals, 22% were self-referrals.

Comments

With one third of the referrals coming from family, friends or self, it is clear that the program has established trust among young people and their parents. Many schools still tend to focus exclusively on "hard busts," where students are caught using drugs or are referred by staff members because of performance problems. These data, however, indicate that referrals really can come from a variety of sources and that different groups tend to be more easily identified and referred through different means. Those who plan

awareness and education events for early-intervention programs should be aware of these tendencies and try to emphasize them when speaking to or writing for different groups. For example, with elementary students it may be helpful to put some emphasis on self-referrals but it would be especially important to provide information to family members to help them refer their elementary-age students for assistance. For senior high students, emphasis on self-referrals would encourage the tendency of older students to come in on their own.

Percentage of boys and girls

Boys made up 49% and girls made up 51% of the referrals to the Minneapolis program.

Comments

The fact that there were almost an equal number of boys and girls in the program should not be misconstrued. Almost one half of the referrals to the Minneapolis Public Schools' Chemical Awareness Program were triggered by problems related to someone else's use of chemicals. When comparing the reasons for referral to the program, we see some marked differences between boys and girls.

General problem categories

The Minneapolis program divides the reasons for referral to the program into four general categories related to drug use:

○ problems related to the student's own use of chemicals, 54%;

○ problems related to someone else's use of chemicals, 42%;

○ problems related to own and other's use, 9% (included in *each* of the two preceding categories);

○ problems not related to chemical use, 13%.

A little more than one half of the referrals, then, were related directly to the drug use of students. Of those with problems related to someone else's use of chemicals, 80% were related to a parent's drug use, 12% to that of siblings, 19% to that of extended family members and 7% to that of friends. Some had problems with more than one drug-using acquaintance. In the 1983-84 school year, statistics were not kept on other problem areas, such as abuse or neglect.

The differences between the reasons for referrals of boys and girls bear close scrutiny. For the boys, 63% were referred for their own use of chemicals and 34.8% were referred for another's use of chemicals. For the girls, 46% were referred for their own use of chemicals and 48.9% were referred for another's use of chemicals. If we look at this issue from another angle, 57% of those referred for their own use were boys and 43% were girls, whereas 40.9% of those referred for another's use were boys and 59.1% were girls.

In senior high school, the difference between boys and girls regarding problems with another's use of chemicals is most marked. Only 15.7% of the senior high school boys in the program came in because of another's use, whereas 34.8% of the girls came in for that reason.

The difference between boys and girls on the own-another's use dichotomy does not show up in the elementary levels. Among elementary children referred to the program, 82.4% of the boys and 82.2% of the girls were sent because of another's use of chemicals.

Comments

The statistics cited in Chapter Three indicate that it is not unreasonable for more boys than girls to be referred to an early-intervention program because of drug use. Boys tend to be involved in the heavier types of drug use and are more likely to act out when they do use drugs. Boys are just as likely as girls, of course, to have an alcoholic or problem-drinking parent. The findings of this program agree with those of other programs: Concerned persons groups typically do serve

many more girls than boys. We need to develop new and better ways to identify or to encourage self-referrals by the male children of alcoholics.

Problem drugs

For students in the Minneapolis early-intervention program, the breakdown on the "chemical most closely associated with the client's problems" was marijuana, 65%; alcohol, 32%; and other drugs, 3%.

Comments

The predominance of marijuana as the most serious drug problem for this population does not necessarily mean that alcohol is not a serious problem for these students. Marijuana appears to be the main problem drug in part because it can be carried easily onto school grounds. This increases the likelihood that students will be caught using marijuana, which, of course, is one of their problems. Alcohol does not cause as many problems in regard to school rules, but it may cause more generalized problems than these statistics indicate. When we look at the Hennepin County Access Unit data in the next chapter, it is obvious that, even with people of the same age, referrals from the schools are much different than referrals from other sources in terms of which drugs were cited as "most problematic."

Related school problems

Figure 9-1 compares the types of problems encountered by students referred for their own drug use and by students referred because of difficulties related to another's use of chemicals.

Comments

Clearly, the school performance of those referred for their own drug use is more markedly affected than those referred because of another's use of drugs. Elementary students, 82% of whom were referred because of a family member's drinking, had the least amount of school problems. Again, if schools were to target for help only those students with the most serious in-school problems, few children of alcoholics who do not have their own drug problems would receive needed services. However, as we have mentioned in preceding chapters, school-related problems are not the only reason, or necessarily the prime reason, for intervening with the children of alcoholics. The incidence of "personal problems unrelated to school performance" is almost as high for the children of alcoholics as it is for those with their own drug use problems. Performance and inner pain are related but not always synchronous. Schools have a great investment in intervening with some of the children of alcoholics on the basis of performance alone, but they have greater reasons for wanting to help this group of young people regardless of the direct connection to school problems.

In-house vs. outside referrals

About two thirds of the referrals made after the school's pre-assessment process received school-based services. The Minneapolis program's pattern of referral was very similar to that of a nearby school district, where two thirds of the referrals generated by the early-intervention program went to in-house services.

The incidence of referral to outside services was lowest among elementary program participants (4.8%), highest among junior high students (48.4%) and mid-range for senior high students (33.9%).

Comments

Whenever possible, the Minneapolis program seems to rely on low-level interventions. Inexpensive, nondisruptive methods and services are used more frequently than the (some-

Figure 9-1 Problems Related to Own or Other's Drug Use

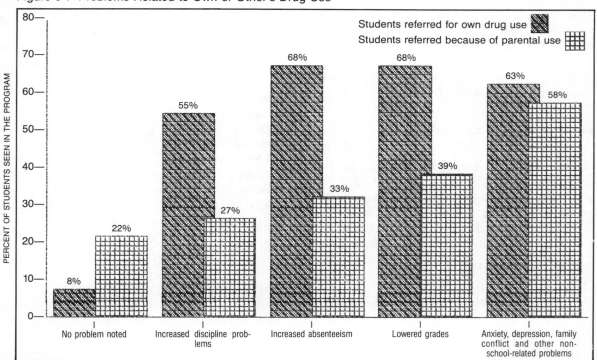

Figure 9-1. The children of alcoholics/drug abusers have fewer problems in school, but they have almost as many non-school-related problems as students who have personal problems with drugs (Minneapolis Public Schools Chemical Awareness Program, 1983/84).

times) more expensive and time-consuming outside services.

Pattern of in-house referrals

The distribution of program participants offered school-based services was as follows. (Percentages refer to the portion of *all students in the program* receiving a particular service.)

○ short-term, one-to-one counseling, 28%;

○ chemical awareness group or class, 25%;

○ Alateen or concerned persons groups, 20%;

○ abstinence support groups, 17%;

○ other services offered by school staff, including special education professionals, social workers and psychologists, 5.6%.

A number of students received more than one referral recommendation. One-to-one counseling, which is limited to six sessions, is most often a route to some other form of service in the school or in the community. Counselors use such sessions to prepare students for a group experience or to support the young person and his or her family as they seek help from community resources.

Pattern of outside referrals

Those referred to services outside the school—about one third of program participants—went to a wide range of different agencies. The percentages below describe the percent *of outside referrals* sent to a particular service (not the percentage of all students in the program sent to a particular service):

○ outpatient treatment for chemical dependency, 21.6%;

○ inpatient treatment for chemical dependency, 17.9%;

○ counseling and family services, 19%;

○ drug-oriented assessment and referral services, 14%;

○ youth service counseling bureau and youth advocacy services, 10.3%;

○ detoxification center, 5.9%;

○ Al-Anon, Alateen and professional services for children of alcoholics, 2.8%;

○ Alcoholics Anonymous, 1.9%;

○ other services, including women's shelters, foster care homes, police, probation officers, medical services, special services for women and inpatient psychiatric treatment, 6.6%.

Comments

It has sometimes been stated that school-based early-intervention programs are simply recruiting grounds for treatment programs. Although these data from the Minneapolis Public Schools cannot refute that statement in terms of the whole country, they can be used to analyze the general issue. Of all the students referred to the program, 13.2% were sent directly to treatment. Drawing on statistics from the next chapter, we estimate that an additional 9.6% of the schools' outside referrals eventually go to treatment via the chemical dependency assessment services or the detoxification units. This adds another 3.2% to the percentage of all the students in the program who go to treatment.

About 16.4% of all the students referred to the program, then, probably end up in treatment. This means that about 0.834% of the entire student body or 1.3% of the secondary student population is referred to treatment annually. Given the amount of heavy and very heavy drug use on school campuses described in Chapter Three, these figures could hardly be considered outrageously high.

Case Examples

To put some flesh on the bones of these statistics, we asked counselors for case examples from their programs. The following examples came from counselors working in the Minneapolis and Mounds View, Minnesota, school districts.

The red eye express

In many programs on drug abuse, educators and others are told to look for bloodshot eyes when screening young people for possible drug use. There are problems with this approach, however. As with any physical symptom, the simple explanation may also be the truth:

Jennifer was referred to a counselor in the drug awareness program because a teacher noticed that she had very red eyes. During the meeting with the counselor, Jennifer said that her eyes had been bothering her and she had just been to the doctor, who prescribed a medication to treat the problem. A quick call to her parents confirmed her story.

This type of referral should probably have gone to the school nurse. Nonetheless, some teachers and others do think of drug problems immediately when they see certain physical symptoms. By treating Jennifer with respect, being open and honest with her parents, while being persistent enough to follow through and confirm her story, the counselor made this a simple matter of screening out and diverting from further review a young person who had one small sign of a drug problem but no corroborating indications.

Embarrassment leads to suspicion

Any adult who is involved in the early-intervention process should be aware of the extreme self-consciousness of some teenagers:

The school nurse referred John to a chemical awareness counselor because of what she considered suspicious behavior. John came to her and said he wanted to leave school because he "didn't feel well," but he would not specify any other symptoms. John looked "funny" to the nurse and she wondered if his eyes looked unusual in some way. When the drug awareness counselor talked with John, he did not have much to say. He admitted that he had not been doing particularly well in school, but the counselor did not press the young man for more information because the interview was going nowhere. She did, however, ask him to have his mother telephone her. When the mother called, she explained that her son had had diarrhea that day and was so embarrassed that he did not want to talk about it. He could not even admit it to the school nurse because of his self-consciousness.

Tough alcoholism counselors may tend to perceive young males as being sly and deceptive rather than, as in this instance, extremely self-conscious and shy. There is always a chance that students may be attempting to cover up embarrassment rather than drug use.

The technique of having the young person tell a parent to call is also part of the early-intervention process. The counselor learns, simply by making that request, whether or not the young person will follow through on commitments.

Guilty until proven innocent

Students who return to school after treatment for chemical dependency sometimes find that they have a reputation to live down:

Fred was suspended by a teacher for acting out in class. She suspected that because he had been in treatment for drug problems, he was using chemicals again. A close review of the situation by the counselor revealed that Fred, who had a learning disability, was having trouble only with the teacher who suspended him. The class also happened to be the one in which Fred's problems with reading and writing were most obvious and he felt miserably inadequate there. There were no indications or reports that Fred had resumed drug use.

Sometimes when young people come out of treatment, they have learned to express their feelings openly and honestly with teachers. Unfortunately, this may be overdone in the classroom, and when students do not swallow their anger, they tend to get in trouble. This was part of the problem that Fred was having in his classes. According to some early-intervention professionals, learning-disabled students tend to present more serious problems after treatment. They tend to be less motivated, to act out more and to apply behavior learned during treatment inappropriately in the classroom setting.

When students in a support group are having trouble with certain teachers, the group facilitator and other group members can encourage them to use the skills they learned in treatment to facilitate clarification of the problems and come to an understanding with the teacher. In many ways, teachers, like parents, think that after a young person comes back from treatment, all the troubles are over and she or he will be perfect from then on. This unreasonable expectation has to be identified as such when it is adversely affecting a student.

Success may be real but unrecognized

In the Introduction we noted that it may be difficult to identify cases of successful early intervention because success means that serious consequences are *avoided* and never given a chance to develop. This may have happened in Sam's case:

Sam was a gifted hockey player who had shown a marked decline in performance since the end of the hockey season. His grades were dropping, he was sleeping in class, he seemed a bit "out of touch" and evasive when questioned by teachers. When the chemical awareness program counselor questioned Sam and investigated the case further, he found little evidence to support the existence of a drug problem but many indications that Sam was depressed and had a medical problem. Apparently Sam had severe allergies. Because he did not like the side effects of the medications, he tended to take them sporadically, which exacerbated their effects. Sam's father, who was at first defensive with and angry at the teacher who referred Sam, also changed his attitude and identified another problem. He realized that Sam should be studying more at night and that he needed

more structure and pressure to study at home. He got that structure and was held more accountable for his time at home in the evening.

Although there was no evidence that Sam was using drugs, it is possible that because he was so depressed and bored he had been using drugs or that he was at least very vulnerable to the attractions of drug use. This intervention, which involved the teachers, the counselor and the parents, may have prevented more serious problems.

Support for a teacher leads to intervention

Sometimes teachers may begin to see a problem with one of their students and take on the responsibility for it. They may believe that if only their presentations were more interesting or more creative, they could hook that student into being excited about the subject:

When one of her students began to seem detached, uninvolved and markedly different from previous semesters, Darlene, a high school math teacher, became concerned. She contacted his parents but did not get any useful information from them. In talking to the school counselors, Darlene said again and again that she felt incompetent, that she could not get through to him and that she should be doing better. The counselors, however, had recently heard about the student from several other teachers and had reliable information, although not hard evidence, that he was using drugs on the school grounds. When the counselors informed Darlene, in general terms, that it was unlikely that the problems were her fault, she felt more confident about expecting him to comply with accepted standards of performance. Eventually he was caught in possession of drugs and successfully referred to treatment.

Simply by giving the teacher feedback that the student appeared to have some kind of problem, that her perceptions were correct and that the problem was not a result of her teaching techniques, the counselors helped Darlene to resume her appropriate role in the early-intervention process: applying fair but strict academic standards.

A parent waiting to be asked

Although school personnel fear hostile reactions from parents whose children seem to be having drug problems, they frequently find parents ready, willing and able to help. Such parents often want to act but do not have the courage, energy or sense of purpose to take the first step:

Billy was manifesting obvious mood swings in his classes. He was very active one day and lethargic the next; he occasionally did excellent work but often did very poorly. When he was feeling "hyper," he would ask to go to the nurse's office frequently, could not pay attention in class and talked openly about using drugs. His grades had slipped. When counselors called his mother to discuss the situation, it became clear that he had an alcohol problem and that she was concerned about it. His problem was considered serious enough to merit outpatient treatment.

In this case, Billy's mother was glad that the early-intervention staff members called, even though she had made no overtures to them. As a single parent, the mother had been confronting the problem alone. Her indecision, rather than denial or hostility, was the reason for the procrastination. The early-intervention program at the school was, quite literally, a lifesaver for her and her son.

Allison helps herself

Those who are just starting an early-intervention program usually find it difficult to believe that young people really come in for help with their own drug problems, but they do:

Allison was already in an Alateen group

because she was having trouble related to her mother's alcoholism. As part of a group exercise one day, she took a 20-question self-assessment screening test on drug use. As a result of her responses, she admitted that she, too, had a drug problem and sought help from the counselor.

Support groups for the children of alcoholics often bring to light young people who are having their own problems with drugs. The fact that the concerned persons or Alateen groups encourage honesty and openness facilitates self-referral.

Friends helping friends

Although young people who have stopped using drugs are encouraged to stay away from friends who still use, they do not always follow this advice. While this can lead to trouble for the young person who is trying to remain drug free, it sometimes works to the benefit of the user:

Barbara had used drugs in the past but had joined an abstinence support group. One morning before school while talking with Mary, a friend who still used drugs, she found out that Mary was having many difficulties in her life because of her drug use. Barbara responded to her friend first by encouraging her to see a counselor and then by accompanying her to the meeting to encourage her to follow through and "come clean." Barbara also supported her friend when she told her parents about her drug use.

Young people in support groups develop confrontation skills that go beyond the perimeter of the group room. Without being preachy or pushy, they frequently find ways to help friends who are still using drugs.

The "hard bust": sometimes the best way to go

With some students, the hard bust, i.e., being caught in possession of a drug or while intoxicated, is the best form of intervention:

It had been clear to his counselors that

Patrick was having problems with drugs. He had talked openly about his drug use, and reliable reports indicated that he was a heavy user in need of help. Since he had been crafty enough not to get caught red-handed and his parents were not cooperative, there was little that could be done. Then one day he was caught while intoxicated on the school grounds. He was sent immediately to a local adolescent detoxification center. This action provided sufficient impetus to prompt the parents to cooperate in formulating a plan for treatment.

Sometimes all the secondary data are in place and waiting to go, but nothing moves until there is concrete evidence of drug use. Although it is seldom medically necessary to send an intoxicated adolescent to a detox center, this was the choice in this case because the counselors wanted the parents to receive a very clear, strong message that Patrick's drug use was a serious issue. Use of the detox center is a way of making an issue out of an incident that might otherwise be swept under the rug and quickly forgotten.

***   ***   ***

In this chapter we looked at the inner workings of a school-based early-intervention program. The decisions made in the school setting are not made in a vacuum, however. How the early-intervention program staff proceeds depends on how outside community services work. In the next chapter we look at the way in which a community assessment service handles cases that have been deemed serious enough to warrant in-depth assessment.

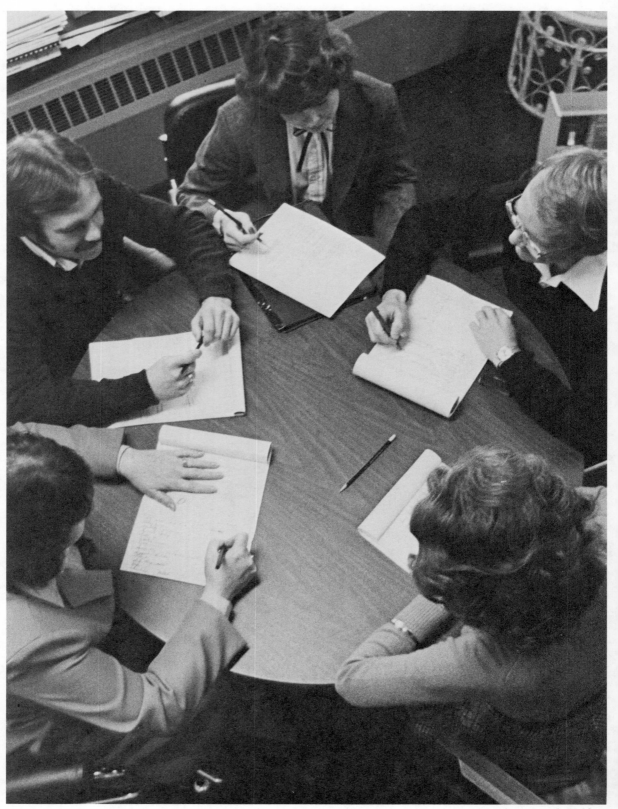

photo: Joseph Muldoon

CHAPTER TEN

PROGRAM ANALYSIS
A Community Assessment Service

Some young people need more help than early-intervention programs in schools or other agencies can provide. Some have chemical problems too serious to even attempt a low-level intervention, and some may run the gamut of early-intervention services to no avail. Others may present such a complex welter of possibly interrelated problems that nothing less than full-scale professional assessment will do. This task falls to community assessment services. They represent the next step after identification, initial action and preliminary assessment.

The County Access Unit

The Hennepin County Access Unit is the public chemical dependency assessment service for the metropolitan Minneapolis area. It offers assessment and referral services to all Hennepin County residents who appear to have problems with alcohol or other drugs. The Access Unit seeks to guide clients to the service that is likely to be most appropriate for their needs and resources. Some clients receive public assistance to pay for services. Staff members see adolescents and adults from every socioeconomic group. Child protection, welfare, court services and other county-sponsored social service agencies use the Access Unit as their primary assessment service for cases involving drug problems. The unit thus serves a greater proportion of young people from public agencies than private assessment services do.

The proportion of adolescents seen at the Access Unit has dropped from 50% ten years ago to 10% in recent years, a shift attributed by the Access Unit staff to the improvement of pre-assessment practices in the schools. Ten years ago, schools tended to send young drug users to the unit without making preliminary assessments of their problems; students caught using for the first time were sent for assessment whether or not there was additional evidence of a serious drug problem. Today the schools use in-house services first, whenever possible. Thus, the cases currently seen at the unit are much more likely to require intensive chemical dependency services than is the general population of drug users.

To demonstrate the workings of this next crucial step after pre-assessment, we consider a sample of 470 young people seen in the Access Unit during a six-month period in 1984. We examine important program statistics: where the young people came from; to what services they were referred; their drug use patterns; and the level of intervention they needed. Then we present 12 case studies showing how the Access Unit staff deals with a range of adolescent drug users.

Statistical Profile of Clients

A statistical overview of the program can provide some insights into the referral patterns for young people who need more service than the schools can offer.

Age of clients

The average age of Access Unit clients in this sample was 16 years—2 years older than the average age of all clients served in the Minneapolis Public Schools' Chemical Awareness Program and 1.2 years older than the average age of secondary school clients.

Comments

This is one indication that the Access Unit deals with drug users whose problems with chemicals are likely to be more advanced and require higher level interventions than the general group of drug users in the Minneapolis Public Schools' Chemical Awareness Program. Those sent to the Access Unit from the school program averaged 15.9 years of age, indicating that they also constitute a different group than the larger group of junior and senior high school clients in the Minneapolis school program. It appears, then, that the schools are being selective in deciding which students are and are not in need of outside referral.

Sex of clients

In the Access Unit, boys made up 55% and girls made up 45% of the client population. This population was slightly different from the school program population, where the male-female ratio was almost even.

Comments

Because the Access Unit is more likely to deal with clients whose problems are related to their own drug use rather than to another's drug problems, it is understandable that more boys than girls would be referred there. As we have said, boys are more likely to be heavier drug users and to act out than girls.

Where they come from

The following list shows the sources of referrals, starting with the most common:

o child protection, welfare, other social services, 25.1%;

o courts, corrections, 21.7%;

o voluntary referrals (self, 5.1%; family, 14.9%; friends, 1.1%), 21.1%;

o school programs, 14.7%;

o detoxification center, 6.2%;

o various chemical dependency services (self-help groups, information and referral agencies, residential and nonresidential treatment programs, halfway houses), 6.1%;

o mental health services, 3.4%;

o medical services, 0.6%.

Comments

Anecdotal reports indicate that many of the self-referrals, family referrals and referrals from friends were influenced by school programs. The referrals from school programs tended to be those made because of "hard busts," i.e., a young person is caught in possession of drugs or while intoxicated. When school personnel have only suspicions or indirect indications that a young person has a serious drug problem, they may not make a direct referral to a community agency, such as the Access Unit, but rather may leave decisions about further action to the parents and the student.

Drug-use patterns

The Hennepin County computerized report forms do not require that the quantity and frequency of drugs used by clients be reported for program data summaries. However, this information is collected on the interview forms. In terms of the "most problematic drug," the Access Unit adolescent population was quite different from the school program population. Alcohol was cited most frequently as the most problematic drug (46.4%), followed closely by marijuana (44.7%). Stimulants were listed as the most problematic drug by only 0.6% of this population; no other drug received notable endorsement. Stimulants were, however, cited as the "third most problematic" drug by 12.3% of the Access Unit population.

Comments

Even in this population of heavier drug users, alcohol and marijuana surpass all other drugs in terms of reported adverse consequences.

Where they went

The following list shows where Access Unit clients were referred, starting with the most frequently used referral options:

o chemical dependency services (nonresidential, 24.5%; residential, 20.6%; other CD services, 6.8%; self-help groups, 3%), 54.9%;

o mental health services, 10.3%;

o child protection, welfare, other social services, 7.2%;

o client at risk, no action taken at this time, 6.8%;

o client not chemically dependent, 6.8%;

o drug education programs, 2.1%;

o medical services, 1.9%;

o courts, corrections, 1.7%;

o client refused referral, 7.3%.

Comments

These statistics can be interpreted only in light of the unique population from which they were derived. Those referred to the unit had already been through some screening process, especially if they came from the schools. This distribution indicates how the group of heavier drug users were dealt with.

Differences between boys and girls

There were few differences between boys and girls in terms of age, racial and ethnic background, court involvement and ranking of most problematic drugs. Significantly more boys (27.3%) had received prior services for chemical dependency than had girls (18.5%). More boys (25.7%) were referred from the courts or corrections services than girls (17%). More girls were referred from mental health services (6.2% for girls, 1.2% for boys) and from child protection, welfare and other social services (32.2% for girls, 18.4% for boys). School referrals were almost the same (15.6% for boys, 15.7% for girls).

There were very few differences in terms of where boys and girls were referred. The most notable difference was, perhaps, that more girls were deemed not to have significant drug problems (8.1%) than boys (3.9%).

Different Populations: Voluntary, School and Court Referrals

To understand how different groups of young people tend to require different types of intervention, we divided the Access Unit statistics into three categories, depending on where clients came from and how they were referred to the unit: voluntary or quasi-voluntary referrals (self, family and friends); school referrals; and referrals from the courts and corrections systems. Court-referred clients tended to be older and male: 64.7% of the court referrals were male and the mean age was 16.3 years. The age and sex distribution of the voluntary and school referrals did not differ significantly from the general Access Unit population.

The following are the major similarities and differences among these groups.

School referrals

School referrals had the most unique drug-use pattern. Among school referrals, marijuana was by far the most problematic drug (68.1%), followed by alcohol (30.4%) and stimulants (15.9%). The other two referral groups, however, cited alcohol as the most problematic drug, followed by marijuana.

Clients referred by schools were also the least likely to have had previous chemical dependency treatment, whereas court-referred clients were the most likely. Only 11.6% of the clients referred to the Access Unit from the schools had had previous services for chemical-use problems, whereas 22% of the voluntary referrals and 26.5% of the court or corrections referrals had. This is an indication that the school programs are providing the earliest intervention service.

Court referrals

Court referrals required higher level interventions. Young people who were referred by the courts tended to have more severe drug and alcohol problems requiring relatively high-level interventions, compared with young people who were referred by schools or who came to the Access Unit voluntarily. In fact, 73.3% of the court-referred clients were referred to some type of chemical dependency service, compared with 50% of the voluntary and school-referred clients. Moreover, 34.3% of the court-referred clients were referred specifically to inpatient treatment, whereas only 15% of the school and voluntary referrals were advised to seek such treatment.

Role of outside services

Mental health and social services play an important role with school referrals. Mental health and social service referrals were made for more than 20% (mental health 14.5%, social service 8.6%) of the young people who came from the schools to the Access Unit. In spite of the relatively high levels of drug use among these students (compared with the general school population and the population of identified drug users in the schools), mental health problems and problems in need of

various social services were still deemed the most important problems for one fifth of these young people. This reinforces the point that drug use is not necessarily the only serious problem in a drug user's life or the first priority for immediate action.

Detoxification Center Referrals

In Chapter Nine, we noted that about 1 of 20 outside referrals made by the schools went to a detoxification center. A review of the referral data from 2020 Adolescent Receiving Center in Minneapolis gives some insights as to the course of action taken with adolescents who enter the system because they were identified as being under the influence of alcohol or other drugs:

o juvenile justice agencies, 15.0%;

o assessment and referral agency, 10.9%;

o other social services, 10.5%;

o mental health program, 4.7%;

o medical services, 0.6%;

o no need for further service, 3.9%;

o self-help groups, 17.8%;

o chemical dependency treatment, inpatient, 29.0%;

o chemical dependency treatment, outpatient, 5.7%;

o aftercare chemical dependency program, 1.2%;

o chemical dependency halfway house, 0.8% (subtotal, all chemical dependency treatment services, 54.5%).

These statistics cover a six-month period in 1984. Like the referrals made by the Access Unit staff, slightly more than one half of the center's referrals went to some type of chemical dependency program.

Case Examples

The remainder of this chapter concerns case examples demonstrating how the Access Unit staff deals with specific types of clients. For each example we describe briefly the reason for the referral; the general pattern of drug use and its consequences; relevant family data and issues; the type of referral made; and the rationale given by the counselor. We also add some general comments on how the example relates to issues discussed elsewhere in this book. Drug use and the related consequences are very important, but they are not the only factors considered during the decision-making process. As these case examples will show, the following issues also come into play in assessment and referral:

■ *Extent of drug use*. This is, of course, still on top of the list for referrals made by the Access Unit. It is the single most important determinant across the board, but it does not stand alone. As part of the process of estimating the severity of a person's drug use, the counselors in the Hennepin County Access Unit are asked to observe which of seven classic "warning signs" of alcoholism or chemical dependency are manifested by the client: increased tolerance, medicinal drinking (e.g., to relieve anxiety or depression), preoccupation with the chemical, drinking alone, blackouts, drinking more than intended and gulping drinks. Two other classic signs, sneaking drinks and hiding a bottle, do not tell us much when applied to an adolescent population, since most adolescents who drink must do so surreptitiously. The counselor uses clinical judgment and does not have to list the specific corroborating data from other parts of the interview form that indicate the presence of these signs.

○ *Relevance of drug use to other problems*. How much does drug use seem to be caused or exacerbated by family problems, school problems or other problems in the person's life? How much does drug use affect other aspects of the person's life? An important factor to determine is whether problems seemed to precede or follow the onset of heavy drug use.

○ *Priority for intervention*. Regardless of what may be defined as the primary problem

or underlying source of the drug problem, the priority for intervention at the time of the interview is a crucial determinant of the immediate course of action.

○ *Obstacles to recovery*. What obstacles make it difficult for this person to improve his or her life by becoming drug free? What can be done to overcome these obstacles?

○ *Personal strengths*. What resources does the person have that could facilitate success in a certain type of program?

○ *Intervention history*. In terms of incremental intervention, has the person had any experiences in low-level interventions? Has the person already been through the entire continuum of care and participated in inpatient treatment?

○ *Motivation or leverage*. Can the probation officer, for instance, limit the person's options to a choice between treatment or incarceration? What influence, if any, does the family have over the young person's preference for treatment?

The following examples illustrate how one community agency handled a number of specific cases. They are intended to be descriptions of how some types of clients are handled, not definitive guidelines for working with all clients. There is seldom only one right referral for an adolescent; but rather, there are a number of options, each of which has certain risks and benefits. For each case, a brief rationale for the referral is given. The reader can critique the referral and the rationale and decide how other referral options may have affected the client in question.

"THEY want me here"

Fifteen-year-old Allen was referred because, according to his parents, he had not been going to school and had failed most of his classes for the past three trimesters. His mother complained that he was sleeping an inordinate amount of time. Consultations between the family and the school truancy officer had culminated in Allen's referral to the Access Unit. Despite his admitting to using a large amount of chemicals, Allen was incensed that his family thought he had a drug problem.

Drug use: Allen started using alcohol at age 12. In eighth grade he used alcohol once or twice every weekend, drinking nearly a six-pack each time. At the time of the interview, he was drinking at least twice every weekend, consuming both beer and hard liquor. He started using marijuana when he was 10 years old and two years later combined marijuana and alcohol use. His sister maintained that he was using before school. He had last used marijuana on the Saturday night prior to the interview, smoking two or three joints at that time.

Allen had also experimented with at least four other types of drugs, including a six-month period of regular use of an inhalant.

Critical incidents: In ninth grade he was caught using drugs on the school grounds.

Prior interventions: Because he was caught using drugs, he attended a chemical awareness class in high school.

Warning signs: The counselor noted evidence of increased tolerance; preoccupation; blackouts (once); gulping drinks; and drinking alcohol and smoking marijuana more than intended on several occasions.

Family history of chemical dependency: No family history of chemical dependency was noted.

General consequences of drug use: Irritability at home and severe school problems were the most marked consequences of his drug use. The onset of school problems occurred in the seventh grade, about two years after he had first experimented with marijuana. He still maintained relationships with some non-drug-using friends, although most of his friends were using drugs.

Relevant family issues: The family was intact, with both parents living at home. The counselor described Allen's mother as the "mediator" in the family and as rather anxious and nervous. The counselor noted that the parents did not really seem to be in touch with their son's drug use and that the responsibility for intervention appeared to have fallen on the sister, who did most of the confronting.

Referral and rationale

Although the client had a very serious drug problem, the parents found it difficult to believe. For that reason the counselor told them that Allen should join a group at school and Alcoholics Anonymous. The counselor wanted to wait several weeks to see if the family could develop more resolve concerning the issue. In the meantime, the client's behavior deteriorated and the parents became more ready to take a stand. When Allen became intoxicated again, his family placed him in an adolescent detox unit and made arrangements for short-term inpatient treatment.

Comments

This very resistant young man needed some controls placed on him. The type of denial and resistance manifested is primitive and basic. Even though his drug use was extreme, he still stated disparagingly in his intake interview, "I'm here because *they* want me here, and they think I'm on dope." He said this just before admitting to heavy weekly and daily drug use. Clearly, there were some family problems, as evidenced by the degree of the parents' denial. Nonetheless, the family was intact and it was likely that a short-term inpatient program could focus the family on the son's drug use and encourage the parents to take control of the situation.

The client had never been involved in a treatment program but had already been in a chemical awareness class. The chemical awareness class did no good whatsoever and the next possible choice could have been outpatient treatment. This may have been a viable option because the family was willing to support treatment and willing to participate. The immaturity of the client and his high degree of denial, however, made it likely that he would attempt to sabotage outpatient treatment by using drugs.

Dishonesty and denial

Seventeen-year-old Brad was referred for evaluation by his family because of problems in the home that appeared to be related to drug use. Brad came to the interview aware of some of the negative consequences of his alcohol and drug use, but he was not ready to give up chemicals. Both his parents and a counselor at a temporary home for runaways believed that some action to stop the drug use was necessary.

Drug use: At the time of the interview, Brad was drinking alcohol regularly on weekends but claimed that he had restricted his use to every other weekend or every third weekend. Marijuana seemed to be his drug of choice. He was smoking marijuana two to three times each day. Other drug use had been minimal. He had experimented with stimulants and tried LSD once but was not currently using these drugs.

Prior interventions: The family had been in family counseling with a psychiatrist for six sessions, but the psychiatrist said therapy should be halted because of Brad's nonparticipation. The client had also broken numerous contracts to abstain from chemical use.

Warning signs: The counselor noted evidence of preoccupation and blackouts.

Family history of chemical dependency: No family history of chemical dependency was noted.

General consequences of drug use: The client had become extremely dishonest. He had stolen from his parents and had become so untrustworthy that they placed a lock on their bedroom door to keep their valuables safe. He had borrowed money from them to purchase a bicycle and spent it on drugs and had, at times, blown his entire paycheck from a part-time job on drugs. He had also been destructive while intoxicated in the home, throwing objects and striking his mother at least once.

The client was at least a half year behind in schoolwork at the time of the interview. He often skipped classes and whole days of school to get high. All of his friends used and

he admitted that he would have to find new friends if he were to stay off drugs.

Relevant family issues: The family was basically intact. He had an older brother who had graduated from high school and joined the Navy.

Referral and rationale

Because the family was still intact and willing to back the referral, the possibility of outpatient treatment was considered. However, because of his occasional violence, the many broken contracts, the parents' inability to place effective controls on his behavior and the fact that all of his friends were drug users, an inpatient program was selected.

Out of control, almost

Fifteen-year-old Connie came to the interview in an extremely resistant and uncooperative mood: "I don't know why I'm here!" Her mother was very passive and did not offer much help during the interview. However, since the client had had several treatment experiences, there was a body of additional information on which to draw.

Drug use: The client had been using alcohol for five years, having started at age 10 while in the fourth grade. She was drinking at least once per month by the time she was 13 years old and, at the time of the interview, had been drinking at least every weekend. She drank beer and hard liquor and would drink between a half and a full pint of hard liquor at a time.

She started using marijuana in the fifth grade and, after some variation over the years, was currently using marijuana and hashish two or three times daily. She had experimented with four other types of drugs but did not use them regularly.

Warning signs: The counselor cited the likelihood of increased tolerance, preoccupation, blackouts, gulping drinks, medicinal drinking and drinking more than intended.

Prior interventions: Connie had been in a detox unit, inpatient evaluation, outpatient treatment and inpatient treatment. She refused to continue outpatient treatment after three weeks and was kicked out of inpatient treatment because of lack of cooperation.

Consequences of drug use: The client had overdosed several times. Her school performance had declined to almost nothing, although she had not formally dropped out of school. Her parents and her sister said that she had undergone a marked personality change since she began her heaviest drug use, changing from a trustworthy to a completely untrustworthy person. Most of her friends were heavy drug users and her closest friend used about as much as she did. Connie had also written bad checks.

Relevant family issues: Her mother and father were divorced and the father had been out of the picture for some time. At the time of the interview, her mother had a boyfriend who was almost totally uninvolved with the girls. The mother was passive and dependent and had completely lost control of her daughter's behavior.

Referral and rationale

The interviewing counselor saw Connie as manipulative, slick, resistant and adept at using treatment language. He saw the mother as a compliant, passive, "lost" woman who had given up her parental prerogatives. She clearly felt incompetent and tended to defend her daughter beyond all reasonable limits. Both the mother and daughter had been physically abused by the mother's boyfriend.

Long-term residential treatment was felt to be the best course of action for several reasons: First, short-term residential treatment had not worked. Second, the mother needed time and a great deal of work to develop the skills needed to offer any kind of direction to her daughters. The long-term residential program that was recommended had a strong family program.

When tough love is too tough

Fifteen-year-old Diane exemplifies the problem of the less manipulative and more

depressed type of adolescent drug user. She came to the interview with her social worker and grandmother.

Drug use: The client had been drinking alcohol for one and one half years and drank very heavily whenever she did drink. She drank the equivalent of 8 to 12 beers each day on the weekend and sometimes drank during the week, as well. She had also been using marijuana for one and one-half years and, just before the time of the interview, had been using marijuana almost constantly, being in a state of intoxication almost 24 hours a day.

She had experimented with minor tranquilizers, stimulants and hallucinogens.

Warning signs: The counselor saw evidence of increased tolerance; preoccupation with drug use; perhaps some blackouts; gulping drinks; medicinal use of marijuana; drinking and using marijuana while alone; and drinking and using more than intended.

Family history of chemical dependency: Both her mother and father and perhaps some of her uncles and grandparents were chemically dependent.

Prior interventions: The client had never received treatment for chemical dependency. She had been in an adolescent day treatment program because of truancy and self-destructive behavior. She had attempted suicide.

General consequences of drug use: Diane had once overdosed on a tranquilizer. She appeared to have little motivation or ability to follow through on any tasks and had changed from a relatively productive student to a constant truant in the year prior to the interview.

Related issues: The family history was extremely chaotic. When Diane was 3½ years old, her mother had abandoned her and her younger sister, leaving them with her father. The father, who was having psychiatric problems, had made numerous suicide attempts. After six years her mother returned but left a month later. Her father subsequently committed suicide. The two young girls were sent to live with their paternal grandparents, who were so old that they were unable to leave the house.

There appeared to be some history of physical or sexual abuse. However, the facts were difficult to determine at the time of the interview.

Diane was generally depressed, feeling lost and hopeless. She felt responsible for the fact that her sister was currently in an adolescent psychiatric unit and that her father had committed suicide. She blamed herself for a great many things over which she had had no control.

Referral and rationale

Diane clearly had a severe problem with chemicals that would interfere with any treatment for depression, sexual problems and other issues. As a complicating factor, however, those issues could also interfere with any primary treatment program for chemical dependency.

The counselor described the ideal program: (1) It should be located outside the city where Diane was living so that she could let go of all the responsibility she felt she had; (2) its duration should not be too short; (3) the grounds of the treatment center should be conducive to her learning to play (she appeared so "grown-up" and was so burdened with responsibility that she had never learned how to play); (4) the program would be able to coordinate Diane's therapy with that of her sister, who was very important to her; (5) the program would provide loving, emotional support; (6) there must be an effective on-site school component.

The client was referred to an adolescent treatment center that strongly emphasized both chemical dependency and psychological issues; she participated in a long-term (three- to six-month) program and an aftercare program.

Comments

Diane's case provides an example of the quiet, depressed type of client that some chemical dependency programs shy away from. She could not be "tough loved" into improving her behavior and saddling her with full responsibility for her problems would have been inappropriate. She had an excessive sense of responsibility and had not had a chance to experience life as a child. However, the high incidence of chemical dependency in her family, coupled with her own heavy drug use, pointed to a clear disposition to chemical dependency and a need to remain completely abstinent from alcohol and other drugs. Some type of warm foster home was probably recommended for her and her sister after treatment. This complex case called for a great deal of coordination between the treatment program, school program, a social worker in the community and probably some psychological service.

A *quick fix for the wrong problem*

Fourteen-year-old Nora came to the Access Unit stating that she needed treatment. Nora had been referred for assessment after seeing a counselor at a teen service for runaways. Prior to the appointment the client had packed her bags and was ready to go to treatment. She seemed very eager to leave her household. Her mother did not know what to do.

Drug use: In seventh grade Nora used alcohol every other weekend and had two or three cans of beer each time. In eighth grade she was drunk once. At the time of the interview, she said she still drank occasionally on weekends. Her marijuana use began at age 12, in the seventh grade. In ninth grade she used almost daily after school. This peak period of pot use lasted for six months but had abated considerably since that time.

The client had experimented with two other drugs, and her brother reported that she had taken lots of over-the-counter stimulants.

Warning signs: The interviewing counselor noted two blackouts, gulping drinks and medicinal drinking.

Family history of chemical dependency: Her father, mother, maternal grandmother and maternal grandfather were all alcoholic.

General consequences of drug use: Consequences noted were very vague. Her mother said that her daughter did not want to be hugged any more, but it was unclear as to whether this was related to current drug use.

Related issues: Her father was an active alcoholic and drank to intoxication two or three days a week. The mother was in what the counselor described as a "long-term, extreme and severe state of co-dependency." The marriage had broken up several times. The mother saw her own defects as the reasons for these breakups and she begged her husband to return home. All members in the family used the mother and scapegoated her. The client was the next most likely scapegoat.

The boyfriend of Nora's best friend had just been in a primary treatment center and, to some extent, it appeared that going to treatment was the "in thing."

Referral and rationale

Counseling at a youth social service agency was recommended, as was family involvement. The family worked on intervention for the father's alcoholism. The interviewing counselor said: "Treatment is a nice quick fix, but what then? Nora is the last member of this family who needs treatment."

Comments

This adolescent from a severely disrupted alcoholic family wanted to use treatment as a way out. She could easily have been labeled "the problem" if she had been sent to primary treatment.

Her OWN plan for treatment

Sixteen-year-old Georgine came to the Access Unit asking for a support group. She said that over the past several months she had been using beer and pot "a couple of times" per week and did not consider herself to be chemically dependent because she was still a teenager. Her social worker had made it Georgine's responsibility to find her own treatment plan.

Drug use: Georgine had been a very heavy user of alcohol. She started when she was 9 years old, and past reports indicated that she blacked out every other time she drank. During her periods of peak use, she was imbibing whiskey four days a week. She started smoking marijuana at age 11 and used heavily, going through many periods of daily use. She had used at least five other drugs and, at times, had injected drugs.

Warning signs: The counselor noted evidence of increased tolerance, blackouts, gulping drinks, medicinal drinking and drinking more than intended.

Prior interventions: The client had had several interventions, both for emotional problems and for chemical dependency.

Family history of chemical dependency: Georgine's mother and two brothers and one of her sisters were chemically dependent. All had gone through treatment within the past three years.

General consequences of drug use: Most of the consequences were not written on the interview form, but there was an attached report. Apparently, Georgine's life was quite chaotic.

Relevant family issues: Georgine's parents were divorced. They had had an emotionally abusive relationship, although no physical abuse took place. Very quiet, subtle and powerful passive-aggressive behavior between them was common. The client had been in a hospital-based youth program at age 12 and a home for delinquent girls at age 15, had been raped at age 12 and had had an abortion.

Referral and rationale

The counselor did "not feel that inpatient treatment would benefit this client at all. She was not ordered to seek treatment, preferred individual counseling and I agree that weekly therapy will focus on expression of feelings and offer the most rewards."

Comments

This referral takes into account two issues regarding decision making: the amount of leverage and/or motivation involved and a consideration of what has already been tried.

This client had been through numerous treatment programs for emotional problems and chemical dependency by the time she reached age 16. She already knew what those programs had to offer and would probably have gained little by going through more treatment while still a teenager. Also, since she was not under court pressure at the time of the interview and did not want to go to treatment, she probably would not have cooperated. The family had no leverage, and school and court authorities were not attempting to use leverage at the time. It is possible that in several years this person may suffer so much that she will decide on her own to cease drug use and join a self-help group. The social service system and continuum of care for chemical dependency had not helped.

A little (more) leverage might suffice

Seventeen-year-old Hal had completed a residential treatment program and had spent time in a halfway house. His parents believed that he was using drugs again and wanted to decide what type of treatment would be most appropriate. Hal had been arrested for forgery and was currently on probation. One stipulation of probation was his abstinence from all drug use.

Drug use: Previous drug use was not reported because this assessment did not concern use prior to treatment. This assessment had only to do with post-treatment use. At the time of the interview, the client was drinking on weekends and sometimes during the week. He usually stopped at six beers but had had as many as 12 beers at a time. The client denied any use of marijuana or any other drugs in the previous month.

General consequences of drug use: Hal's parents did not speak of any marked change in his behavior, but because of past problems with chemicals they were very concerned about any drug use at all.

Relevant family issues: Hal was currently living with his parents. He had a brother aged 22 and a sister aged 32. One older brother would have been 35 years old had he lived. The counselor thought that the client may have had lingering concerns surrounding the death of his brother. The counselor also noted that the mother seemed to be overbearing and that Hal may have been having trouble with this.

The interview was quite chaotic. Hal's mother talked almost incessantly and had a difficult time focusing on his alcohol and drug history. She frequently digressed to things that had happened in the past. The client had trouble finding an opportunity to speak because his mother dominated the interview. The father tended to sit back, tried to make his wife speak more to the point and waited for opportunities to make his thoughts known.

Referral and rationale

Hal admitted using chemicals since he had completed treatment. His probation officer explained the legal consequences of continued use, and Hal said he understood. Hal also said that he would like to work on some personal issues with a counselor. The recommended plan called for him to undergo counseling and to expect that pressure from the probation officer and parents would take care of current drug use. The counselor thought that the major problem with this family was the apparent lack of communication between the mother and the father as to what they expected from their son. The client was playing one parent against the other, with some success. The parents also apparently had their own unresolved relationship problems. The client was referred for personal counseling at a social service agency.

Comments

This client had already undergone treatment for chemical dependency, and it was hoped that the leverage of a concerned probation officer and the parents would be sufficient to deal with drug use at the time. An interesting aspect of this referral is that family systems work was not recommended. The primary client, Hal, was the youngest of three children. The others were fully independent adults and this 17-year-old client would soon be on his own as well. Had this client been the oldest in the family, with younger children still living at home, more pressure may have been placed on the parents to work on family problems.

The risk of low-level intervention

Seventeen-year-old Paul felt that his troubles with authority and rules were more serious than his problem with chemicals. It appeared that conflict with his stepmother had precipitated his referral to the Access Unit.

Drug use: Paul had first tried alcohol at age 13 and currently was drinking five to six beers once or twice a week. He had been using marijuana since age 14 and was currently using about one joint every other day. His use had declined somewhat since his sophomore year, when he was using twice daily. He said his marijuana use at school declined because he wanted to avoid the consequences of being caught in school.

Warning signs: The counselor noted evidence of increased tolerance and drinking alone.

General consequences of drug use: The client had never been apprehended for a drug-related violation, although he had sometimes driven while intoxicated. His mother said that his temper was more volatile when he used, that he was more blunt about his feelings and that his motivation had decreased. His father saw him as listless.

Paul's grades were Cs and Ds in junior and senior high school. In tenth grade, when his drug use was at its worst, he skipped classes to get high.

Relevant family issues: Paul was living at home with his father and stepmother. His older sister was not living at home. He fought openly with his stepmother and frequently called his mother and stepfather in Nebraska to play them against his father and stepmother.

Referral and rationale

Paul was referred to a drug education class in the high school. He had had no prior chemical dependency treatment or drug education, and the counselor felt that his drug use could be affected by a low-level intervention. If his problems continued, an outpatient drug program with a strong emphasis on family issues would be the next appropriate step.

The counselor also believed that clear guidelines were needed if he planned to continue living in his stepmother's home. If he chose to ignore the guidelines, he should be asked to leave and begin making a life for himself.

Comments

This listless, semi-depressed or perhaps very depressed young man undoubtedly has some issues other than drug use in his life that call for counseling. Since the drug use itself was not life-threatening at this point, the low-level intervention, i.e., drug education, was an appropriate response. Outpatient drug treatment may very well become necessary for this young man. One danger of the low-level intervention is that Paul may not do well and, after he turns 18 and leaves school, will be under less pressure to seek help and ineligible for school-based services.

An encourageable "incorrigible"

Sixteen-year-old John had been ordered by the court to have an alcohol-drug assessment after his parents filed a petition to have him declared incorrigible. The client stated at the beginning, "The only time I get high is when there are problems at home." He did not believe his chemical use was a problem.

Drug use: John said he drank alcohol "once in a while" but usually had a negative reaction to it. He drank alcohol at keggers. He had last imbibed three weeks prior to the interview. Marijuana was his drug of choice. He had been smoking it for the past year and said that he used it one to two times a week and "whenever a major skirmish happens at home." He had gone through a period of daily drug use several months before the interview.

The client had done very little experimenting with other drugs, having used stimulants and hallucinogens on only one or two occasions.

Family history of chemical dependency: His father was an alcoholic and attended Alcoholics Anonymous. His maternal uncle was also an alcoholic.

General consequences of drug use: The major consequences seemed to be related to trouble at home, such as violating curfew. His mother had filed a petition to have him declared incorrigible and John had appeared in juvenile court.

Relevant family issues: John had a 19-year-old sister, a 12-year-old half brother, a 6-year-old half sister and a 19-year-old cousin. The client was having problems with his older sister, who also had a 1-year-old child. He did not get along with his stepfather, who had been married to his mother for ten years.

Referral and rationale

The client and his mother and stepfather were advised to attend a drug education program offered by a community service agency. The education program focused on family issues as well as drugs.

Comments

This client had never been involved in any counseling, drug education program or treatment. During the interview he behaved appropriately enough and, given the leverage that the court had over him, he was willing enough to cooperate. He still seemed to have a viable relationship with his mother, although there was some distance between them. For this reason, a low-level intervention, i.e., drug education, had some potential for success.

First things first?

Seventeen-year-old Kevin had a history of being absent from home and was currently under a court order to have an assessment. He did not feel that his chemical use was a primary problem.

Drug use: Kevin said that he did not care for alcohol and drank rarely, not more than once a month. In the previous year he had used marijuana two and, sometimes, three times a week. He had occasionally gotten high before going to school.

Family history of chemical dependency: Kevin's mother and a paternal uncle were alcoholics.

Previous interventions: The client was once recommended for inpatient treatment but did not have the funds to pay for it. He was also asked to participate in a residential treatment program in another setting but did not go.

General consequences of drug use: The client admitted to selling some possessions to get money to buy marijuana. The parents attributed the client's having quit a job and his inability to get another to drug use.

Relevant family issues: Kevin was currently living with his father and stepmother. Three stepchildren were still living at home.

The counselor said that the client was facing a number of pressing psychological issues: his parents were divorced and his mother lived in California; his mother apparently was chemically dependent and had custody of his younger sister and brother; his mother had a boyfriend who was also chemically dependent and had been physically abusive to her and verbally abusive toward her children. The client wished to protect them, but he was 1,800 miles away. Kevin's father had remarried and his stepmother brought three of her children (aged 15, 20 and 22) with her. The client did not have a room of his own and felt that he was an outsider in the family.

Referral and rationale

The Access Unit counselor recommended therapy for Kevin, to be coordinated by his social worker; family counseling was also recommended.

The counselor saw Kevin's drug use as secondary to the many important emotional and family issues in his life. Key factors precipitating his drug use were the separation of his parents; the stepfamily issues; the frustrated need to protect his mother and siblings; and his mother's chemical dependency and generally unhealthy relationships with men.

Comments

This client clearly had emotional problems that needed to be resolved, but there was a risk in this referral. If the client's drug use continued, it may well have interfered with any attempts at therapy.

Establishing controls over problem behavior

Fourteen-year-old Linda was referred to a county social worker when her mother petitioned the court to have her declared incorrigible. The social worker brought her to the Hennepin County Access Unit. Linda did not believe she had a problem with alcohol and drugs. It was her psychologist who suggested that Linda have her drug use assessed.

Drug use: Linda drank alcohol every weekend. She said she liked to "get wasted" when she drank. The client also smoked marijuana with other people four times per week but never bought her own. She said she did not know how much she smoked each time. She had experimented briefly with two other drugs.

Family history of problematic use: Many of Linda's cousins, aunts and uncles got drunk frequently.

General consequences of drug use: When Linda was high, she became verbally aggressive. Her mother believed that her daughter's drug use had affected their relationship.

Relevant family issues: Linda, an only child, was currently living with her mother. Her father had left when she was 3 years old and had maintained little contact. She and her mother did not get along well. Linda had not been attending school; she came and went as she pleased, kept late hours and slept late into the morning. Most of her friends used alcohol and drugs.

Referral and rationale

The Access Unit counselor recommended an intense behavior modification program provided by the adolescent treatment program of a psychiatric unit. Although Linda acknowledged heavy binge use of chemicals, the counselor felt that chemical use was a manifestation of her general character disorder and behavioral problems. She had a history of shoplifting, running away and other problems that preceded her drug use. She was sexually active and presented herself generally as a tough, streetwise kid. Her mother was totally unable to control the situation and had been for some time.

No support for change

Seventeen-year-old Michael came to the Access Unit at the request of his probation officer. He had been picked up with his older brother, who had burglarized a store.

Drug use: Michael started using alcohol when he was 14 or 15 years old and had been using it occasionally for about two and one half years. No other drug use was noted.

General consequences of drug use: No consequences directly related to drug use were uncovered.

Family history of chemical dependency: Michael's mother and stepfather were alcoholics but denied having any current problems with alcohol. His father was also an alcoholic.

Relevant family issues: Michael's family was severely disrupted. His father was alcoholic and physically abusive. He also had some legal problems. The older brother admitted that he instigated the burglary and that he had occasionally given his younger brother something to drink. He said that he did not believe his brother drank very much.

Referral and rationale

The client did not admit to having any serious problems with chemicals, and none of his family indicated that he had any problems.

The counselor's intuitive feeling was that, although Michael's drug use was probably more serious than others were willing to admit, it probably was not the major determinant of the young man's problems at the time. The extremely chaotic, unstructured family life also militated against any focused drug treatment program since there would be little support for this young person in treatment.

The major recommendation was that Michael work with a social worker who could help him make decisions concerning vocational development and find a better place to live.

***   ***   ***

Having seen how some programs work with young drug users, we will change our focus. The next chapter provides a format for readers to assess how their own schools or agencies work with young drug users.

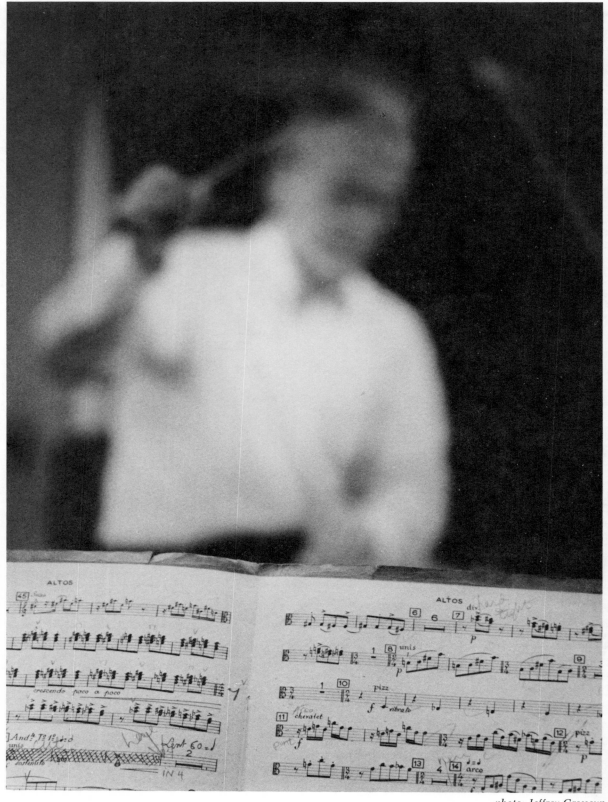

photo: Jeffrey Grosscup

CHAPTER ELEVEN

PROGRAM REVIEW
Back to the Basics

The evaluation of early-intervention programs can take any number of forms, from informal meetings with students, faculty and advisory board members to the collection and analysis of very specific data on clients and program flow. We suggest that early-intervention program staff members plan and evaluate their programs by comparing current functioning and future plans with the six basic processes of early intervention: identification, initial action, preliminary assessment, referral to appropriate resources, appropriate use of an adequate continuum of care in the community and support for change. When people use these processes to set goals and then relate these goals to specific program activities they have made a giant step toward coherent planning, implementation and evaluation. They also have developed a means of resolving disagreements in a consistent and rational fashion.

There is sometimes a one-to-one relationship between a goal and a program activity. An assessment interview with a student, for instance, contributes primarily, though not exclusively, to the program goal of providing *preliminary assessment* services. We say "not exclusively" because the competence and fairness of the counselor performing the interview will become known to other students

and have an impact on the willingness of staff members and students to take positive *initial action* regarding a drug or other problem. Such activities as community outreach, on the other hand, can contribute to a wide variety of goals, depending on the need the outreach event has been designed to meet. In the early stages of program development, for instance, most educational sessions for staff members, students and parents focus on drug and other personal problems. They will also attempt to explain the nature of program services and how to go about taking advantage of the services. This, obviously, contributes to the goals of identification and initial action. At a later stage in program development, when more and more students are attempting to remain drug free, outreach events can focus on the positive aspects of drug-free living and on the idea that young people have a right not to be pressured into using drugs at every party or school event they attend. This contributes to the sixth goal of early-intervention programs, i.e., providing support for personal changes.

In this chapter we offer a format for beginning the evaluation process, a structured format of inquiry that can serve immediately in discussions about a program as well as in the development of formal data-gathering practices. We look at each of the six processes in detail, consider the common barriers to the smooth functioning of each process, describe how the activities in an early-intervention program relate to it and consider some evaluation questions relevant to the process.

Identification

For the most part, early-intervention program services are first offered to those young people with the most serious drug problems, but schools and service agencies eventually find it productive to provide certain services to the children of alcoholics and to those whose personal problems put them at a high risk for drug use. Most programs eventually provide the means to:

o identify young people whose use of mood-altering chemicals is affecting or likely to affect their academic performance, general school behavior, health and emotional development;

o identify young people whose personal problems—including but not limited to the use of mood-altering chemicals—are affecting or likely to affect their academic performance, general school behavior, health and emotional development; and

o identify people whose lives are being harmfully affected by the chemical use of a family member or friend.

Problems may be identified by the person with the problem, by a staff member, by a friend, by a relative or by any other concerned person. Although a decline in academic performance and violations of school regulations commonly bring students to the attention of school personnel, many of those in need of services would be neglected if these behavioral patterns were the only criteria for identification and referral. Some young people can perform quite well while using drugs or while having very serious problems with alcoholic parents. As we have noted, the best way to maximize the potential of a program

is to develop all possible means of problem identification.

Barriers to identification

A general lack of awareness
Whenever we ask those currently working with adolescents to name barriers most likely to keep them from reaching young people in need, lack of awareness of drug problems always ranks high on the list.

Implications for programming: Well-planned awareness and education programs are essential. During the process of community mobilization to establish programs against drug abuse, awareness and education programs can remain very general, aimed primarily at getting people to realize the scope of the drug problem and its impact on the community. As early-intervention programs begin to develop, however, awareness and education programs should become more focused. Certain groups—parents, coaches, alternative-school staff, probation officers, social workers, nurses and others—must learn how the specific segment of the student, court-referred or patient population they work with tends to avoid identification and initial action on drug problems; they must also learn how to circumvent those avoidance techniques. Awareness and education must continue year-round and evolve from year to year.

Lack of criteria for acceptable performance
When young people are not held to clear standards of performance and behavior, drug-related declines in performance go unnoticed. As a result, many chances to reach young people in need may be missed.

Implications for programming: Early-intervention programs affect and are affected by the school or agency in which they work. If a school or a particular program in that school has lower standards for performance, drug use is less likely to be identified. The early-intervention program staff should support efforts to apply clear, consistent academic and behavioral standards to all students.

Starting with the wrong concept of the drug problem

If people choose to see drug abuse not as a serious health problem but rather as merely the negative behavior of a group of "losers," they may find it difficult to see and accept the fact that many of the "good" kids whom they like are also having problems with drugs. They need the right concepts before they can acquire the right percepts. This is also true of problems other than drug use and chemical dependency.

Implications for programming: In drawing up policy statements and designing awareness programs, program staff members must be careful about the way they conceptualize the drug problem. The concepts presented in Chapters Two and Three can serve as guidelines. For example, the fact that there is a broad range of drug use problems, touching all groups of young people in schools, courts and social service agencies, should be made clear to keep people from stereotyping drug users. In court populations, the incidence of very heavy drug use may be so high that less heavy use starts to look normal to the staff. Even daily use of marijuana may seem less of a problem when use of more dangerous drugs, such as amphetamines, PCP, cocaine and heroin, is not uncommon among the population being served. We want people to stop seeing drug use as normal behavior, but we also do not want them to look on it as a moral failing or as a sure sign of an antisocial personality.

Clear policy and procedural statements also help in the identification of young people in need by making it known that drug abuse problems are considered an important issue. By defining drug abuse as a "serious health problem" or chemical dependency as a "disease," a school, court or social service agency has culled certain behaviors from the general, unquestioned activities of young people and made them a focus of concern. When these behaviors are made an issue for discussion, pressure for resolution has begun.

Overlooking some groups

Specific groups may have less chance of being identified. Some people allow athletes to slip through the system because "a little drinking is normal for a jock." Also, minority students are sometimes missed because staff members tend to perceive their problems as "behavioral" rather than as related to chemical dependency or emotional issues.

Implications for programming: Some groups will inevitably be overlooked during program development. Sometimes such oversight is built into the system, as when all referrals to a program come through the disciplinary process. Sometimes it is simply because one of the key counselors prefers to work with a certain type of young person. Constant review of who is being identified and consideration of how to change procedures to identify those being overlooked are essential aspects of program evolution.

Looking only for acute drug effects

In the past it was suggested that teachers and probation officers could best help the process of early intervention by learning to detect the signs of acute drug abuse (e.g., red eyes, slurred speech). This approach has its place in an early-intervention program, but it is useful only if the proper context has been created for a broader system of identification, referral and assistance.

Implications for programming: In some communities, the approach of looking for signs of drug abuse has been pushed so hard that when people first hear of the early-intervention program, they *presume* that it focuses exclusively on apprehending intoxicated or hung over young people. This misconception must be dealt with directly in awareness and education programs.

Goal Setting Is Often Discredited

Time and again it has been demonstrated that the successful people in top management are those who can establish meaningful organizational goals and integrate those goals into the daily activities of the organization. Nevertheless, the idea of developing a careful, goal-oriented planning process has often been written off as irrelevant by people in social services. Some reasons for their discrediting the goal-oriented approach are:

○ *Goals are not used.* Goal setting is often presented as a process done merely to appease a compulsive bureaucracy, and often it is. Many goal statements have been written, accepted with a smile and placed in the files with no consideration of the possibility that they could truly affect the nature of the organization.

○ *The "MMM effect."* Many talks about goal setting are extremely mechanistic. A great deal of emphasis is placed on specifically defined terms. Minute distinctions are made among primary, long-range, ultimate, secondary, intermediate, formal and informal goals. Such terms as "methods," "tasks," "activities" and "steps" may imply distinct levels of operation or they may be used more loosely. The use of such terms is helpful if and only if the goals and goal-setting process deal with issues relevant to the people who must attain those goals. Otherwise, goals, objectives and activities all become a meaningless, mechanistic morass (MMM).

○ *The predominance of ideology.* Often, no practical distinction is made between program goals and program philosophy. In such cases, program philosophy becomes a heart-felt ideology. Any program results that are not compatible with the ideology are ignored. The goals, then, become totally irrelevant.

There *is* a big difference between program goals and program philosophy, but many of us fail to see the distinction. Goals help us specify what we want to *do* and everything subsumed under that goal may specify how much of it we want to do, who we want to help do it and when tasks must be completed.

Philosophy has to do with all of our *assumptions* about adolescents, about the issues of drug use and abuse, about schools, about parents, about teachers and about all the various other issues that help guide decisions. All of the assumptions we make form the belief system that, if accepted by most people in the organization, becomes the program philosophy.

In a healthy organization or program, the goals, program philosophy and program evaluation form a three-part system of checks and balances. If we do not establish verifiable program goals, then our assumptions about adolescents and about drugs are never confirmed or ruled out. The philosophy becomes immutable ideology.

Program review questions

1. Whom do you really want to serve? Just the drug users who get caught? Those who have performance problems that do not respond to normal academic procedures? Those affected by parental alcoholism?

2. What information do you have concerning the need for services among the young people in your school or agency? Where can that information be found? Who must be contacted in order for that information to be made available?

3. Whom are you currently identifying? Does this pattern of identification appear to be close to the number and types of young people actually in need?

4. What biases are apparent in your identification process? Are these biases acceptable for the time being or must they be changed immediately?

5. How are cases currently being identified? Are there patterns that you want to change? Are there different techniques, such as those mentioned in this book, that you would want to employ?

6. Which of the barriers to identification presented in this book are manifested in your school or agency? What other barriers to identification are there among the school or agency staff? Among the young people in need? Among their friends? Among their parents? Among the staff of the early-intervention program itself?

7. Are you confusing barriers to identification with barriers to initial action? Do people already know who is using drugs and who is probably being abused at home, but are not acting on this information? If so, do not waste time teaching people to identify problems; rather, teach them what to *do* about those problems.

8. Are you being passive in identifying those in need of service? Is this acceptable for the time being? Are you already serving all the cases you can handle given the current resources?

9. Do you want to change your data recording system to keep better track of who is being identified?

10. What can you do immediately to improve the identification process? What can you do in the next several weeks or months to improve the process? What can you do in the next year?

Initial Action

Once a teacher, drug user, friend, parent, probation officer or social worker has noticed behavior that may indicate a problem with drugs, the goal is to take *some* positive action. People must be aware of how to take the first, crucial step toward resolution of the problem, and that first step must be fairly simple and convenient. The important point is to break down the tendency toward inertia. In school programs, a concerned person could take one of the following actions:

- *Clarify*. A teacher, coach, counselor, administrator or other adult in the school can talk to the student, not to counsel but to clarify the situation.

- *Consult*. The staff member can request a consultation or advice from a person knowledgeable about the early-intervention program and the issues of chemical dependency.

- *Refer*. The staff member can make a referral to the early-intervention program, requesting an in-house preliminary assessment.

The way in which these initial actions are prioritized and conducted depends on procedures. Some school programs in the early stages of development send most students through administrative channels first, because of disciplinary problems. Other programs have been able to motivate a large number of students to come into the program through self-referrals or referrals from family or friends.

The possibility of positive action being taken by a friend or directly by a troubled student, client or probationer should not be discounted as an unrealistic dream. Everything possible should be done to facilitate self-referrals or requests for information and assistance by users or their friends. If this avenue of action is taken seriously by the program staff, then young people also take it seriously.

Barriers to initial action

Inappropriate counseling

Some staff members prefer to counsel young people directly. This can be a process that teachers enjoy and do not want to give up in favor of early referral. In some instances, such one-to-one counseling can be beneficial for a time. Sometimes, however, attempts to comfort, advise or show understanding do little to move the young person toward resolution of the problem.

Concern about labeling or diagnosis

A staff member may feel that a diagnosis is necessary before referring a person for preliminary assessment. Many people believe they have to know exactly what the problem is before they take any action at all. Others may be afraid that if they refer a person, he or she will automatically be labeled chemically dependent, a bad kid or a druggie.

Implications for programming: Experience in employee assistance programs has shown that when supervisors felt they had to counsel their employees or diagnose their problems, they were less likely to refer employees for help. They spent too much time either trying to figure out the situation themselves or worrying that if they got involved they would be taking on more than they could handle. When people know that they do not have to diagnose or solve problems and that some simple observations are sufficient for an appropriate referral, they are more likely to make an early referral. This does not mean that teachers should not discuss an academic problem with the parents and the student first. If the school normally operates in this manner, an early-intervention program should not override these procedures.

Lack of trust

Students and staff members may not trust the program. If, in the past, students have simply been expelled for any issue related to drug use, people may be reluctant to deal with drug problems. If staff members and students do not believe that they can share concerns with a counselor without the administration finding out, they are less likely to seek assistance.

Implications for programming: Trust is the most important factor in motivating people to act on problems once those problems have been identified—trust that the family or student will not be prejudged or labeled, trust that competent preliminary assessment will be available; trust that the services used by the school will be helpful; trust that students and staff members will not be looked down on for using the program. Negative or misleading rumors about the program must be identified and countered.

Confidentiality is a crucial issue here. It should be made clear that there are appropriate safeguards for students' rights and that confidentiality will be protected. Personal information about a student or her or his family gathered during the preliminary assessment for drug or other personal problems must not be placed in the student's cumulative records. Administrators and teachers who are not members of the early-intervention program staff should not have automatic, direct access to that information. All program staff members must be trained to follow guidelines for professional conduct regarding confidentiality. In a court setting, admission of drug use should rarely, if ever, be used to file further charges against a young person or to have his or her friends arrested.

Lack of administrative backup

Staff members may be afraid that administrators will not back them up if they confront a student. If, in the past, some angry and defensive parents attacked teachers and those teachers were not defended by the administration, all staff members may be reluctant to take action.

Implications for programming: Just as administrative support is crucial in the early stages of program development, it continues to be necessary throughout the program's existence. If, for example, an administrator overlooks the transgressions of a couple of star athletes, trust in the program will be severely harmed.

Unclear policies and procedures

Staff members or students may not understand the nature of the policies, procedures and services of the program and may not know whom to contact. If a school has inadequately defined or inconsistently applied policies and procedures regarding drug use, it is more difficult to confront students who are using drugs.

Implications for programming: A simple, clear procedural statement coupled with brief training on those procedures solves many problems in this area. Clear guidelines for referral are necessary. The early-intervention program staff should draw up procedural statements specific to various work areas or school buildings. Policies can be general, but procedures must relate to each staff member's duties. Teachers, for example, use different procedures for referral than school nurses.

Program review questions

1. What barriers to initial action exist in your school or agency? What barriers exist among staff members, young people, administrators, parents and others?

2. Have you been confusing problems in identification with problems in initial action? Do staff members understand the distinction?

3. Have you considered the hidden personal agendas that may be barriers to initial action? Some staff members may intellectualize about the technicalities of program methods to cover fears about drug use, family problems and abuse (in their own lives as well as in the lives of others). These fears must be addressed in a caring, nonjudgmental manner.

4. Are some staff members willing to act in certain cases but not in others? What distinctions are being made and what can be done about this?

5. Are teachers clarifying problem situations with students, seeking consultation when necessary and referring appropriately? Do people tend to refer too early, too late or not at all?

6. What types of awareness programs need to be conducted with specific groups to increase the number of appropriate initial responses to problem situations? What information, encouragement and support must be communicated?

7. Have there been any changes in the patterns of initial action in the last several weeks or months? Have these changes been positive or negative? What has caused the change?

8. What data do you have regarding initial action (number of referrals to the program, number of requests for consultation, anecdotal reports from individuals)?

9. What can you do to collect more data about the number and type of initial actions being made by people in your school or agency?

10. What can you do immediately to improve program functioning related to initial action? What can you do in the next several weeks or months? What can you do in the next year?

Preliminary Assessment

The type of in-house preliminary assessment performed depends, to a large extent, on the services available in the school or agency and in the community. The goal of the preliminary assessment is not to provide an in-depth description of people and their problems but rather to gather the minimum amount of information needed to come to one of the following conclusions:

○ No special action must be taken regarding drug or other personal problems. Regular school, agency or court procedures should be followed.

○ The person may have some problems, but further monitoring in the school setting is needed. A time for a review of the situation may also be specified.

○ The person has some problems for which present in-house services may suffice; they should be tried first.

○ Referral to an outside agency for an in-depth assessment of drug or other personal problems and possible treatment is warranted.

The process of *motivating* is tightly intertwined with the preliminary assessment process. When a young person is made aware of the full impact of his or her actions and when the options are clear and specific, he or she is likely to be more motivated to change behavior.

Barriers to preliminary assessment

Lack of specific data

In many schools and agencies, young people are referred to counselors with a note describing some vague complaint rather than specific data. This lack of data hampers the ability of those performing the preliminary assessment. They may have to base their judgments strictly on clinical observations, reports from the young clients and reports from parents who may or may not be entirely cooperative.

Implications for programming: The use of a standard data-gathering form can help the preliminary assessment process. Assessment should not be viewed as a clinical process that takes place in a counselor's office. Observations of student behavior in the classroom, in the locker room, on the playing field and at social events are crucial to the process. To meet this need, the early-intervention program staff can provide simple systems for the gathering and assessment of information re-

lated to a particular student. The in-house assessors must define their boundaries and understand that they will usually perform only the initial steps of assessment and intervention, not complete the process.

Limited referral options

A lack of effective support services in the school or agency and a lack of in-depth assessment and treatment services in the community can make the preliminary assessment meaningless. We want to assess not only the person but the options available to the person as well. Some communities have little to offer to adolescents with drug use and related problems.

Implications for programming: Schools, courts and social services may have to hire or contract with their own highly trained assessment person until community services catch up. They may also have to encourage community agencies to be more responsive to adolescent problems by demonstrating a clear need for assessment, counseling and treatment services. It is actually quite common for early-intervention services to develop more rapidly than the various treatment services. In such cases, young people may have to travel some distance, even out of state, to obtain necessary treatment. This practical solution helps deal with the most urgent cases until local services can develop.

Lack of cooperation on the part of parents and their children

For preliminary assessment to work at its best, especially if the assessment must take place over time, cooperation on the part of parents and young people is essential. If, for instance, the assessment involves having the young person attend a three-week Insight Group to learn more about his or her relationship with chemicals, the process is worthless if the young person does not attend. It can also be severely hampered if parents do not cooperate by insisting on a curfew and on a drug-free lifestyle during the assessment period. The same is true if the school recommends in-depth assessment by a community agency and parents choose to ignore this recommendation.

Implications for programming: Firm and consistent application of policies is crucial to motivate young people and parents, who might otherwise expect the usual second chance. The school does not have to threaten to expel each student but can make it clear that if the person's behavior does not improve, restrictions will result. Fairness is also essential. When parents feel their children are not being singled out, they are more likely to cooperate. Awareness and education projects can be extremely helpful in making all parents aware of the program and in showing them that the program offers effective help to young people and their families. Then, when parents are contacted concerning a child's drug use, they are prepared for the possibility of drug problems and may be more willing to cooperate with early-intervention program services.

Program review questions

1. Is the process of preliminary assessment clearly defined? Is it broken down into steps: consultation on referrals, data gathering, review of the data, student interviews, meeting with parents, use of Insight Groups for assessment, post-group review and decision making?

2. Have responsibilities for different steps in the preliminary assessment process been delegated? Is everyone clear about who is to do what when?

3. Is the system too structured, sufficiently structured or too informal?

4. Are problems with the preliminary assessment clearly differentiated from problems with the continuum of care? When the only service for drug problems is chemical dependency treatment, for instance, assessors find themselves in a situation that makes assessment very difficult.

5. Do all staff members understand the limits of the preliminary assessment process? Are

some staff members making the task too hard by trying to make assessment too comprehensive or too definitive?

6. What types of training and awareness programs are needed to increase the ability of teachers, parents and others to gather and pass on information that will be useful in the preliminary assessment and referral process?

7. What kind of data-gathering system is needed to assess the functioning of the preliminary assessment process? Are the current records helpful in any way? Is there a way to review the assessment method to discover how to standardize and improve it?

8. What can you do immediately to improve the preliminary assessment process? What can you do in the next several weeks or months? In the next year?

Referral to and Appropriate Use of the Continuum of Care

The mechanisms of referral from an early-intervention program are directly under the control of the program staff. The range and quality of the continuum of services for drug abuse can be influenced, but not controlled, by the staff of an early-intervention program. Although referral and use of the continuum of care are two different processes, they overlap so much in practice that the barriers to and facilitators of these processes are often one and the same.

Many students or juvenile offenders have problems that in-house services, such as education and awareness groups, can help solve. Others need counseling or more in-depth treatment. Schools, courts and social service agencies can legitimately offer a number of in-house services, including educational programs about drugs, their effects and other issues; short-term counseling and group sessions for developing personal awareness of how such issues are affecting one's life; and support groups for young people who want to stay free from chemicals or to work on other issues in their lives. Existing community services can also play important roles in school-based early-intervention programs. Volunteers from community agencies can serve on advisory boards, help in community outreach activities and function as support group facilitators.

Early-intervention programs need some guidelines for making referrals. Criteria for referrals to specific agencies should be established through discussions between the program staff and the staff of each agency involved. Guidelines for referral should be written and patterns of referral studied carefully to determine how consistent program staff members have been in sending people for additional help and how consistent community service providers have been in accepting or rejecting referrals.

Follow-up is an important part of improving the referral process. The best follow-up involves at least two stages. The first involves ascertaining through phone calls or written communication, whether or not the referral was appropriate. This should be done fairly early, perhaps a week after a young person has begun to participate in a program. The second stage involves contacting the client after she or he has completed the course of treatment or counseling to find out her or his opinions of the service and whether the service appears to have been helpful. A possible third stage of follow-up involves finding out whether or not the service actually changed the attitudes and behavior or contributed to the general well-being of the client. This type of follow-up involves a certain amount of scientific rigor that goes beyond the resources of most early-intervention programs and usually calls for an infusion of grant money targeted for such a purpose.

Barriers

Lack of in-house support services or lack of staff cooperation
Some coordinators of school drug programs have developed effective support groups for

students but continually run into difficulty with staff members or administrators who do not want to take the trouble to adjust students' schedules so that they can attend such groups. As a result, many students whose problems are not very serious have to be referred to service providers outside the school.

Implications for programming: In-service training must be offered to the staff to make them aware of the benefits of certain in-house services and to gain their cooperation in helping students who must alter their schedules to take advantage of such services. When these problems are addressed, administrative backup is essential.

Lack of familiarity with community services
This is a major impediment to making appropriate referrals.

Implications for programming: Familiarity with community services must be developed. People working with an early-intervention program must identify those community agencies most appropriate to handle the problems likely to be presented by young drug users. They must also clarify criteria for admission and treatment, such as cost, age, sex and geographical location.

Poor communication
Lack of communication or cooperation between service agencies and the schools or courts makes it difficult to exchange the kind of information needed not only to refer a young person to an agency but also to assist that agency with its job and to help the young person when he or she returns.

Implications for programming: Schools and courts must work hard to establish healthy relationships with community agencies. This means not only having good informal connections but also establishing methods of transferring data that are acceptable to the school, parents, students and agency.

Gaps in the continuum of care or barriers to service
If needed services are not available in the

community, it is difficult to use the continuum of care effectively. Community agencies that charge more for their services than the parents can afford can create a serious problem.

Implications for programming: Schools, courts and other early-intervention agencies should let service providers know about the emerging needs of their students and offer suggestions about the development of new services. State and private service providers should be constantly made aware of young people who are not receiving adequate service because they do not have adequate insurance.

Difficult cases referred too soon

Some young people have multiple problems and thus do not fit well in any one setting. There may be temptation to move them out of the school or court system quickly. Instead of benefiting from a series of appropriate referrals, they tend to get dumped from one system to another.

Implications for programming: Schools and community agencies must learn to share the responsibility for helping to alleviate drug problems. The "dumping" of difficult cases is not an uncommon practice in the field of mental health and chemical dependency. Some mental health centers do not want to deal with chemical problems and simply refer chemically dependent clients to an alcoholism treatment center. Likewise, when alcoholics are found to also be schizophrenic, some chemical dependency counselors prefer to transfer them to the mental health system. Such dumping can also happen among parents, schools and social service agencies. A child who has severe discipline problems and also uses drugs should not be sent to a chemical dependency treatment center in the hope that such treatment will cure the discipline problems.

Program review questions

1. Are the basic community services in place and available to all young people in your school or agency?

2. Are some important services lacking? Do some service providers purport to be competent in dealing with adolescents but are only competent in working with adults? What can be done about this?

3. Are there any major barriers to getting help from specific agencies, such as insurance issues, the working hours of service providers or the unwillingness of some agencies to work with certain clients? What can be done about these barriers?

4. One important way to improve the continuum of care is for early-intervention programs to clearly demonstrate the need for service, thus motivating further community action. Is your school or agency accumulating data on the unmet needs of young people?

5. Has the early-intervention program staff leaned toward or away from using certain counseling or treatment modalities? Does the bias concern the general nature of the service or stem from problems with a specific agency that provides that service? For example, is no one being referred to a local hospital because the early-intervention staff does not believe in inpatient treatment or because they think the counselors there are incompetent?

6. What can your staff do to improve its ability to make appropriate referrals? Do you need some simple tools, such as a list of all the appropriate agencies along with information about types of service and hours of service?

7. What communication barriers exist between the school or agency staff and the various service providers in the community?

8. Is there a clear understanding regarding the issue of client confidentiality? Does everyone understand what type of release forms are needed to share information about clients?

9. When you refer a young person, do you have any way of knowing whether the client ever reached the service recommended? Do you have any way of knowing whether the referral was appropriate and whether the client derived any benefit from the service provided?

10. What can you do immediately to improve the referral process and general use of the continuum of care? What can you do in the next several weeks or months? In the next year?

Support for Personal Changes

Some simple assistance provided in schools, court services and social service agencies can be invaluable to young people who are trying to stop their drug use or who want to do something about difficulties arising from living with drug or alcohol abusers. Many treatment center counselors have said that they began to have significant success with adolescents when schools began offering post-treatment support services to students. Too often the concept of support groups or support services is loosely defined, leaving staff members to conceptualize needs and address problems in an idiosyncratic fashion. Support services can, however, be conceptualized and implemented in a methodical fashion subject to review and revision.

Barriers to support

Peer pressure
Peer pressure in the school is one of the biggest barriers to staying drug free.

Implications for programming: The general school climate has a strong effect on the success of early-intervention efforts. When it is generally considered appropriate to abstain from drug use and to ask others to do the same, these norms help prevent drug use and help support those who have already been in trouble with drugs and are trying to change their lives for the better. The early-intervention program staff is as responsible as, but no more responsible than, other school or agency staff members for developing such a climate.

The period of transition from drug use to no use
For those who have left the school or community for inpatient treatment, the shock of returning can be exceptionally difficult.

Implications for programming: All adults involved with young drug users should be aware of the stresses involved in making the transition from relying on drugs to not using them at all. Some of the problems are "technical" and would be trying to anyone: scheduling classes, making up for lost time, getting credit for work done while in treatment and trying to fit a support group into an already crowded class schedule. A young person returning from treatment has a special need for the guidance of an adult who knows and can manipulate the various systems in the school and the community.

Schools can also help by providing inexpensive services compatible with the school setting. These can be provided as needed. For example, if there are three or four students returning from inpatient treatment, the school could start an aftercare group; if a number of children of alcoholics have been identified, a concerned persons group could be developed.

Remember that support groups offered by the school are different than aftercare groups offered by treatment centers. Part of the purpose of treatment-oriented aftercare groups is to encourage further work on the many personal and family issues uncovered in treatment. The purpose of school-sponsored aftercare groups is to lend support in fending off pressures to use drugs and for developing strategies for building drug-free lifestyles. They focus on helping the young person navigate through an environment in which the many forces that may have contributed to the original pattern of drug use are still at play.

Staff hostility
Hostility from teachers and other staff members, in reaction to the actions of the student

before the drug use stopped, is another barrier to providing support.

Implications for programming: This issue must be raised and dealt with during staff in-service training. The early-intervention program staff must be ready to work with individual teachers, probation officers, police and judges who might be extremely prejudiced by the behavior a young person exhibited prior to the intervention for drug or other personal problems.

Program review questions

1. Is the term "support" used in a specific manner? Is there a distinction, for instance, between "support groups" for young people who have decided to stop using drugs and "support groups" for students who have just been confronted with their drug use?

2. Are support services geared only to young people who have completed treatment? Are services needed for those who have not gone through treatment?

3. Are support groups and other support services being undermined by problems in scheduling and by a general lack of cooperation on the part of teachers and other adults?

4. For students coming back from treatment the period immediately following reentry is especially difficult. Are there special provisions for helping these young people at this particular time?

5. Is the general school and community environment so drug-laden that young people face an overwhelming task when trying to remain drug free? If so, what can the early-intervention program staff do to lessen the general level of drug use in the community?

6. Is your school or agency taking on too much of the burden in regard to support services? Can other service providers be enlisted to help? What can be done to start more support services and to coordinate them with your students' or clients' needs?

7. What can you do immediately to improve support services for young people? What can you do in the next several weeks or months? In the next year?

***   ***   ***

The primary purpose of this chapter has been to review basic concepts and clarify generic goals that apply to all early-intervention programs, whether they are operating in schools, juvenile justice agencies or any other community institution or agency.

Keep these early-intervention processes in mind whenever undertaking any organizational task or talking with any group. If you are talking to a group of teachers, parents or students, ask yourself:

○ How can this group of people help the program in terms of the process of identification of problems?

○ How do their skills or roles in the school relate to the assessment process?

○ How can they help us improve referral procedures, develop more referral options and get the most out of community services?

○ How can they help provide a more supportive environment for students who want to make changes?

Whenever there is a disagreement over prioritizing a task in terms of time or money, try to see how that task is relevant to a specific process of early intervention.

CREATIVITY AND INNOVATION

Will the Circle Be Unbroken?

Our journey, dear reader, has been long and, occasionally, arduous. The challenges we face concerning adolescent drug use and related problems are neither simple to comprehend nor easy to address. Books that attempt to facilitate understanding and action in this area are bound to take the reader over rocky ground and up steep grades.

If you have read the preceding chapters and taken some time for reflection, if you jotted down an idea or two that came to mind while reading or if you have made plans for starting or changing a program, then your efforts here have been of value. Whatever time you spend in critical thought and careful planning will save much more time in the field, when you are working with young people and their families.

A person who has read this far has been given a considerable number of concepts and an abundance of information that can serve as food for creative thought. Many of the program ideas suggested here were new to readers and will serve as stepping stones to newer, more creative ideas. But creativity, cherish it though we do, is only part of the recipe. Creativity put into *action* brings *innovation*, new ways of doing things, not just new ways of thinking about things. When innovations are tested in the real world and problems are confronted and resolved, further creative thinking and innovation are possible. The growth of ideas and effective programming, then, is circular and mutually enhancing. We offer this book to people with the hope that they will use the information, comment on it and develop new ways of solving the problems we have addressed. We would like, in five years, to publish the second edition of this book with your own ideas, programming concepts and research integrated into it.

Go well. Via con Dios. Shalom.

Appendixes

Insight Groups

In Chapter Seven we described the general function of an Insight Group in the overall process of early intervention. Here we outline a typical Insight Group format.

Sample Insight Group Format

Insight Groups do not have a copyrighted format devised by one agency or publishing company. They have been developed by a wide range of contributors. Since they are still evolving, the outline provided here is only an example—a descriptive rather than a prescriptive example—of this process.

Optional materials

In some schools and court settings the Insight Group programs have developed assignment books consisting of a variety of exercises copied or derived from prevention programs and self-awareness publications. Since these books are used for classroom purposes only and are not distributed to people outside the school building or group setting, such use *appears* to be compatible with current copyright regulations. Some systems have developed simple self-assessment questionnaires based on published material but altered in various ways to meet the needs of the population served by the group. Some assignment books have paper and pencil exercises that have been altered and passed around so often that they are probably in the public domain.

In many programs, printed assignment books are not used. Facilitators plan their exercises according to the goals of each session but do not require that participants bring in assignments completed at home. In place of the self-assessment questionnaires, a facilitator meets with participants individually before or early in the Insight Group cycle. The facilitator asks a number of questions concerning drug use, not to complete a definitive assessment of the person's relationship with chemicals but to form some hypotheses about how the young person might function in the Insight Group and what Insight methods could be emphasized to help the person get the most out of the process. Sample questions that help this Insight-focused assessment follow this outline.

Facilitators

Most young people sent to an Insight Group are difficult to deal with because they are angry about being required to attend the group and defensive about their feelings and their drug use. For this and other reasons, it is useful to have two or more facilitators. One makes the formal presentation of didactic material; the other person or persons observe the group members closely, looking for any behavioral signs that may provide insights into a person's feelings and serve as springboards for discussion after the formal presentation. As one counselor put it, "We don't wait for people to open up. We look for cues and then ask them what they think about some of the material. We also go in loaded with data from the forms teachers have filled out and the drug use assessment the kid has gone through with a facilitator. These data can help us expand on the information presented in the formal presentations. Having more facilitators makes it more likely that one of us will remember and relate the data to the class."

Insight Group Summary

The typical format consists of nine one-hour sessions held during a three-week period.

Young people can join a group only at the beginning of a nine-session cycle.

Session 1: Orientation

Rules and regulations are reviewed and expectations clarified. The structure of the Insight Group cycle is described and the necessity for punctual attendance at *all* sessions is stressed. Since the cycle is not open-ended, participants cannot simply make up a session they miss by attending that particular session in the next cycle. The nine-session cycle must be taken as a whole and in sequence. If participants miss a single session, they must repeat the entire cycle.

Goals of the Insight Group are described, and the facilitator emphasizes that this is an opportunity for the participants to begin a process of self-assessment.

Confidentiality is discussed. Facilitators who participate in self-help groups may have trouble when they begin an Insight Group. Unlike a self-help group participant, a facilitator in a school-based Insight Group cannot say, "Everything in this group is confidential and nothing leaves this group." If a young person appears to be in a life-threatening situation, for instance, that information must be brought to the attention of his or her parents. Usually, as trust develops in the group, participants are willing to have the facilitators assist them in discussing their drug problems with their parents. The discussion of confidentiality in Appendix B is relevant to the Insight Group process.

In this first session, participants begin to ventilate their anger about being referred to the group and discuss the incidents that led to their referral. The facilitators do not necessarily confront blatant rationalization or denial in this session. The participants are given two clear messages. First, they learn that they can be open with their feelings of anger and frustration and will not be punished for expressing them. Second, they learn that despite their feelings of being the victims of a grave injustice, they will be expected to follow procedures.

Participants are, then, provided with a very visible, comprehensible structure that specifies expectations for behavior, describes the hoped-for goals of the group and offers tools to help them benefit from a variety of learning activities. Manipulation by the participants is minimized because the process leaves little room for maneuvering.

Contracts concerning abstinence

If a participant has entered the Insight Group through the school's disciplinary process, most likely she or he will already have made some type of contract to remain free from chemicals. Such contracts should not be viewed as deeply felt personal commitments. Since the participants are often quite angry and rebellious when they sign the contracts, they most likely have no intention of keeping them. Disciplinary contracts usually involve a statement that expresses the expectation that the young person will not use chemicals because it is against school regulations and state laws. The statement also spells out specific consequences for any violations. Such contracts can be viewed as affirmations that authorities have been very clear with the young people who sign them and that there is no deception on either side. Both sides know exactly what the expectations are and what the consequences of deviating from those expectations will be.

A contract made with a school counselor or with a group is quite different. If a person has grown to like and trust the facilitator and the other group members and he or she makes a *personal* commitment to remain free from chemicals, that is a real commitment to abstinence. This type of group commitment need not come during the first session of the Insight Group cycle but can be put off until some trust develops within the group. This does not mean that the group acquiesces to drug use. It simply indicates that a commitment to the group is meaningless until the group forms some sort of cohesive spirit.

Session 2: Progression of drug use

Participants finish explaining their reasons for being in the group. The formal presentation for this session concerns the progression of drug use from experimentation to regular use to harmful involvement to complete dependency. Many schools and court services use the concept of chemical dependency as their main model for serious drug problems. Although it is likely that the incidence of psychological dependence on drugs is higher among the participants in an Insight Group than in the general population of young people, facilitators cannot presume that all participants are alcoholic or chemically dependent. Emphasis here remains on *both* the acute and the possible chronic effects of drug use. Participants in an Insight Group, especially in the early stages of the process, tend to feel very judged if they are labeled. Any additional labeling other than that inherent in their inclusion in the group is likely to make them feel more shamed and more defensive.

If written self-assessment questionnaires have been used, the facilitator should peruse this material before the third session begins. If they have not been used, the one-to-one interviews should be finished before the third session begins. The material derived from these Insight-based assessments is used to determine the general tone of the group and the type of interventions that will be needed for individuals and for the group as a whole.

Session 3: Feelings

A "feeling chart" is often used here to describe the relationship between feelings and drug use or dependency. It is made clear that alcohol is a drug and that "chemical" abuse or dependency refers to the use of all mood-altering chemicals—legal or illegal, prescribed or not prescribed. The ways in which drugs mask or blunt natural feelings are discussed. In discussing these issues, facilitators often use examples from the data collected from self-assessment questionnaires or one-to-one interviews. Confidentiality is maintained, however, and the person on whose behavior an example is based is not identified by the facilitator. Although specific participants are not named, this material has a very powerful effect when young people see how their own behavior relates to the broader issues presented.

This session is a turning point for many participants. They begin to open up, offer their own examples of feelings and defenses and become more actively involved in the session as the information presented hits home. The facilitators are no longer seen as people who are there to confront them or accuse them of "bad" behavior but as people who seem to evince some empathy. Facilitators also have to be prepared for participants who, when they start seeing the group as less of a punishment and more of a personal approach that is likely to touch their feelings, become frightened, defensive, quiet or hostile. Facilitators need to validate their feelings, allow participants to have them and avoid making judgments. With luck, these participants will, as the group progresses, develop the capacity to see themselves in the material presented rather than simply listen to the interpretations of facilitators.

I'll Quit Tomorrow by Vernon Johnson contains information relevant to this session.

Session 4: Defenses

The facilitator lists and gives examples of the most commonly used defenses: denial, rationalization, minimization, projection, and others. The facilitators emphasize that defenses are often unconscious and closely related to low self-esteem. Such books as *Why Am I Afraid to Tell You Who I Am?* by John Powell are used as resources for this session. A list of feelings can also be compiled by the group.

The Johari Window

This is a popular exercise used in a variety of educational and training events. The "window" describes four levels of awareness or lack of awareness: "things I know about myself that others also know"; "things that I know that others don't know"; "things about myself that I am not aware of but others are"; and "things about myself that neither I nor others are aware of." The Johari Window is made real to participants by asking them questions about what they keep hidden in their lives, what they do not tell their friends, what they may or may not be able to admit, even to themselves, and so forth. Participants are not expected to answer all these questions openly; they are asked to think about them. One group facilitator who uses this technique said, "I never cease to be amazed at the power of this particular presentation. I have watched kids quiet down in this session because we touch something in them. I can see it. Their sense of isolation and loneliness is very strong."

A detailed description of a Johari Window group exercise is given in *The 1973 Annual Handbook for Group Facilitators* (Pfeiffer and Jones, 1973).

Session 5: Role play on defenses

This session begins with a continuation of material from the previous session. Facilitators can ask participants how their drug-using behavior relates to the Johari Window. After the input relevant to the Johari concepts has been completed, some role plays that demonstrate how defenses work in real life can be tried. In a school setting, facilitators can play the roles of a student, an assistant principal and the parents. They act out a mini-intervention session held in the assistant principal's office. In a court setting, of course, the roles of judge, probation officer and parents can be used.

Participants observe, describe and discuss the defenses acted out in the role plays. Humor frequently pervades this session. Participants laugh, not only at the facilitators' acting skills but also at themselves as they see their own behaviors mimicked. When they see some of their defenses portrayed, kids of-

ten say things like, "Boy, I really use that one on my own mother, that silent treatment."

Session 6: Role play on defenses and giving helpful feedback

If there are still some role plays that would benefit the group, they can be completed at the beginning of this session. Of course, a review of the basic concepts of defenses would help to remind participants of what these role plays really mean. The rest of the session can be spent in discussing and demonstrating the skills of listening and giving helpful feedback. This prepares participants for the next session, in which some group discussion and confrontation about the drug use of the participants will take place. Techniques such as clarifying an issue before responding, using nonjudgmental terms, sticking to specific statements and using "I-statements" (taking personal responsibility for one's feelings and beliefs) are all part of the repertoire of useful confrontation techniques. *The Skilled Helper* by Gerard Egan offers some useful guidelines for "effective challenging."

It is fairly easy to demonstrate through humorous role play that clumsy and judgmental confrontations with parents, teachers or friends are counterproductive. This session prepares the group for smoother operation in Session 7.

Session 7: Confrontation

The Insight interview described later in this appendix contains questions that are often used to prepare young people to participate in Insight Groups. Although the actual interviews are more free flowing than the question-by-question format of the assessment sheet indicates, the structured sheet can be useful in this session. The facilitators can discuss the implications of some of the questions and emphasize responses that reveal serious symptoms, such as blackouts. Participants can be encouraged to discuss their own responses and, depending upon the climate that has developed in the group, may confront one another. Participants should be allowed to confront one another openly only if the facilitators feel that it will be a positive process.

Remember that the question sheet is not a diagnostic assessment of chemical use history; it is simply a way to motivate a person to start thinking about problems related to drugs. For example, a participant can answer the question "Have you received any negative feedback about your drug use?" with a simple "no." However, the question may prompt the person to remember instances of negative feedback and to consider what they mean for his or her relationships and what they imply about his or her drug use.

Session 8: Outside resources

A recovering chemically dependent person—possibly a former participant in the Insight Group—may be invited to speak about outside resources. Professionals from community agencies can also address the group.

One of the most important tasks to accomplish in this session on outside resources is to review the important issues that are often related to drug abuse among teenagers: parental alcoholism; family violence or family problems in general; sexual abuse; divorce, death and separation; and concerns about sexual identity. It need not be implied that these problems are more prevalent among Insight Group participants than among the general population. Participants can merely be given the message that the counselors are not shocked by these problems and are open to hearing about people's concerns in these areas. Participants also learn that specific resources outside the school and court can help kids with these problems.

Session 9: Evaluation and commitment

Participants receive feedback from facilitators and other group members and are assigned a facilitator for a 30-day follow-up.

Participants can also be given a resource book that provides the locations and times of Alcoholics Anonymous, Alateen and Families Anonymous meetings along with the names and addresses of appropriate social service agencies in their area.

Insight Interview

Authors' note: *Mike Andert wrote the following portion of the appendix. Mike is a teacher at Minnetonka, Minnesota, Senior High School and has been active in Minnetonka's Student Assistance Core Team for the past seven years. During that time, Mike facilitated many Insight Groups. The practical approach he presents here was developed as he worked with adolescent students.*

Minnetonka is a suburban high school that serves about 2,000 students in grades 9 through 12. The students with whom Mike works are referred to the Insight Group from a variety of sources. Most referrals come from the high school administration as a response to violations of the school's chemical use policy. Referrals also come from parents, police officers, teachers and others.

Mike has developed an exercise found to be very helpful as an introduction to the Insight Group process. Called the Insight interview, it has been used successfully by Mike and others at Minnetonka Senior High School as part of the difficult task of helping adolescents look at their chemical use via the Insight Group.

By Mike Andert

I have found the Insight interview to be helpful for orientating new participants to an Insight Group. This awareness activity includes an exploration of the participant's recent chemical use. I ask students a series of questions, much like those employed in a drug use evaluation, not simply in an attempt to gather data but to help students begin to look at their relationship with chemicals and to help them become aware of any denial they may have around their chemical use.

I always conduct these interviews outside the group, soon after a participant has been referred to the Insight Group. The interview gives me, as the group facilitator, an opportunity to discuss group rules and objectives and to begin to establish a trusting relationship with the new member. I must be able to confront the participant when there is evidence of denial, but I must do so in a supportive way.

Supportive confrontation can be a difficult technique to employ. The following example illustrates the dynamic. Bill, age 16, was referred to our Insight Group because he was caught using alcohol during a school activity. During the Insight interview, Bill described the many arguments he had had with his mother. He related that she frequently berated him for drinking. He claimed that she had unfairly grounded him more than once, and he felt that his relationship with his mother "couldn't get much worse." Helping Bill see the connection between his drinking behavior and his failing relationship with his mother is an example of a supportive confrontation.

This supportive confrontation began with me asking him some questions about the incident for which he was grounded. How many times had similar incidents happened before? Does his mother ground him just to have a sense of power over him or is she concerned about his welfare? Is she concerned specifically about his drinking? What other things has Bill been doing that she doesn't like?

Helping Bill form a coherent overview of his and his mother's situation helped a great deal. I made sure not to label him and didn't ask him to consider whether his mother was mad at him because "he is a drunk" but, rather, whether his mother was concerned about drinking and the dangers it causes. When I made a summary statement, it was in the form of a hypothesis for Bill to consider: "Is it possible that your mother's concern has grown out of the many different times your drinking has caused problems for you? Is it possible that the real source of her anger and frustration is your drinking behavior?" Since the interview preceded the Insight Group, I didn't need answers to these questions. I simply let it go and asked the questions in several different ways during the group process that followed.

During an Insight interview, I begin to communicate many of the group norms or conditions under which the Insight Group operates. One of the first norms I try to set in an Insight Group is to give participants permission to talk about their chemical use in a way that is neither judgmental nor clouded by delusion. I find the Insight interview to be an opportune setting for me to model this kind of behavior. Introducing the activity to the adolescent, I try to explain clearly that the interview is intended to raise awareness, not gather data. If I'm successful in modeling this behavior, the adolescent finds it easier to adopt.

I'm continually aware of the risk that adolescents take by talking to me, an adult, about their chemical use. As a group facilitator, I need to recognize this risk and affirm that it is being taken. Any feedback must be given out of the concern I feel for the young person with whom I'm working. I also need to remember that if I rush to give advice or a recommendation about the need for counseling or treatment, it may simply make the person feel labeled.

The Insight interview is best done on a one-to-one basis. At least one and one half hours are needed to complete the activity. It has not proved successful to split the exercise into two blocks of time. Most adolescents are not put off by my taking notes and it is helpful to refer to them during the interview. I've found that offering to show the notes to the participant at the end of the session has relieved some of her or his fear. It has not proved successful to simply hand the questions out to adolescents, ask them to read them and fill in the answers.

Confidentiality

At the beginning of the Insight interview I tell the young person that if certain facts lead me to fear for his or her immediate health and safety, I may have to reveal that information to others. I also say that I won't surprise the person by making calls or referrals without his or her knowledge.

Adolescents need to understand that the interview is *not* an evaluation. They need to know that any information or awareness that comes out of this activity is theirs as well as mine. Most important, they need to feel that this process will not be harmful. My reaction to specific details revealed during the Insight interview affects their willingness to share in the Insight Group.

Perhaps the toughest decision any Insight Group facilitator can be confronted with is how to handle data indicating that the person needs more help than an Insight Group can provide. My experience with adolescents in Insight Groups has taught me that information shared "for me only," or information that "can't leave the room," can lead to a difficult bind. Mary is a case in point.

Mary, age 15, was referred to our Insight Group by her parents because they found a small amount of marijuana in her room. Her parents were also concerned about her recent change in friends and her moodiness. During the Insight interview, Mary admitted that she was getting high nearly every day and had tried to cut down or quit a number of times but couldn't. She was afraid she "might become dependent" but was adamant that she didn't want her parents to find out.

Intervention is a process, and in Mary's case, since she was much more involved with chemicals than anyone had suspected, the process had jumped from beginning to end, with no time spent in the middle. In my opinion, Mary needed treatment, not an Insight Group. As the facilitator, I needed to act. Mary needed to share with her parents the extent of her involvement with chemicals. As it turned out, Mary was able to do this. If she had been unwilling or unable, I would have needed to act in Mary's best interest by talking with her parents myself, even over Mary's objections.

In our school, those referred to the Insight Group are young people with a relatively low level of chemical use experience. Those with more significant chemical problems are more likely to skip the Insight Group and go directly to a more advanced stage of intervention. Thus, the Insight interviews we conduct tend to be with adolescents who have less denial and delusion than I would expect to see in young people in the treatment setting.

The Insight Group facilitator must be sensitive to an adolescent's level of denial. During an Insight interview, it may be very apparent that the student is not willing to see a connection between use, abuse and harmful consequences or may even be unwilling to participate in the interview. In this situation, I find it best to deal solely with the chemical problem that resulted in the referral. If, as the young person moves through the Insight Group process, more chemical use data are revealed, I may be able to confront the denial.

Interview questions

The order of the questions may be altered to fit the situation. Generally, the questions that are easier for the young person to talk about come first. As the adolescent and the facilitator spend more time with the questions, rapport builds and the person may eventually be willing to answer questions that seemed too threatening early in the interview. Thus, some of the questions may appear to be repetitious. If a question has been thoroughly answered and discussed, it need not be asked again. Of course, I use many more clarifying questions than I have indicated in this list.

1. What kinds of chemicals, including alcohol, do you or have you used?

2. When did you first begin using?

3. Tell me what the words "drunk" or "high" mean to you. How often do you get drunk or high?

Note: Questions 1, 2 and 3 are asked simply to gather facts. I start asking about chemical-related issues at the beginning of the interview because, most often, chemical use is the issue that brought the adolescent and me together. In another context, it may not be appropriate to start off asking about drug use. If a student comes to me after class and mentions some vague problems that he or she is having at school or at home, I do not focus on drugs immediately. In the pre-Insight Group context, however, drug use has already been raised as a crucial issue—most often because the student has violated the school's code on chemical use or possession—and the student expects to discuss the issue.

4. Do your parents know you use? What happened when they first found out? How did you feel about them finding out?

5. Of the people you know, how many use? How many of your close friends use? Are you concerned about their use?

6. How much do your parents use? Brothers? Sisters? Are you concerned about their use?

7. If you're concerned about a friend's or family member's use, have you ever told him or her that?

Note: Questions 4 through 7 introduce the idea of consequences related to use by asking about others' concerns about the participant's use. The idea that negative consequences encompass more than being physically sick will be new to many adolescents. These questions also help depict the general milieu in which a person's drug use takes place. It may be that among his or her friends or even within his or her family, drug use is implicitly or explicitly accepted.

8. How do you get your chemicals?

Note: Question 8 can lead to surprising candidness. The adolescent's response can serve as a measure of how much trust has been established. This question may be more revealing in some areas of the country than in others. In some school districts, for instance, young people are sufficiently affluent and the norm of sharing drugs is so well entrenched that kids do not have to work very hard to get chemicals. In other areas, everyone is more or less expected to pay for her or his own stash. If a person is working very hard and spending a lot of time trying to keep a supply of alcohol and other drugs, that tells you more than if a person uses only the drugs that come his way, like manna from heaven.

9. If you were to pay for all the chemicals you used in the past month, how much would you have spent?

Note: Question 9 usually indicates a high degree of minimizing. Cost factors vary with the chemicals used and geographic location.

10. Has anyone ever told you that you use too much? How did that make you feel?

11. Think about the people you hung around with before you started to use. Do you still see them? If you don't, is it because they don't use or don't use as much as you?

12. Do you work? Ever use before or at work? Ever had any problems with chemicals at work?

Note: Questions 10, 11 and 12 deal with consequences. I try to help the adolescent get in touch with any feelings about the consequences that come to light.

13. Have you ever been busted (home, school, police)? Should you have been?

Note: If a student has been referred to the Insight Group specifically because of a drug-related violation, the details come out in response to question 13. I try to sense whether or not I am dealing with a naive person who may not be too harmfully involved and simply was not slick enough to avoid apprehension. Often, this type of student readily admits that the problem is his or her own fault. The more harmfully involved student is more likely to boast about the many times he or she has used and could have been busted yet complain bitterly that he or she got busted this time because of a "nosy assistant principal who just hangs around the bathrooms trying to catch kids."

14. When do you like to use?

15. Do you ever use before or during school? How does it affect your performance in school?

16. How did you do in school in _____ (grade prior to start of use)?

17. How is school going for you now (grades, attendance, friends)?

18. Does it take more, less or about the same to get high or drunk?

19. Tell me what you think the difference is between blacking out and passing out. Ever do either?

Note: Blackouts are typical "red flags" in a chemical use evaluation. I very seldom find an adolescent who blacks out, but this may merely reflect the particular population of adolescents I see.

20. Are you sexually active? When high or drunk?

21. How do you keep people from finding out that you use? How does it make you feel to do that?

Note: Questions 20 and 21 can often put adolescents in touch with their shame. If you pursue this issue gently, it's possible to help adolescents begin to look at how their chemical use may be affecting their value system.

22. Where do you keep your stash?

Note: Question 22 is another question that provides a sense of how much trust has been established during the interview. If the student gives a very specific answer, you have some indication that you are building trust and a solid rapport with her or him.

23. Tell me what you think a rule about drug use would be. Do you have any?

24. Have you ever broken one of your own rules? How did you feel?

25. What's it like when you use alone? How does it feel?

26. Have you ever tried to quit? Why? How did it go?

27. Is it as much fun to use now as it used to be?

Note: Questions 23 through 27 ask participants to look at various rules regarding drug use. Of most importance is helping them see that they do follow some self-imposed guidelines, such as never using during the school day and never getting drunk during the week. A discussion about how many rules they have and how well they follow them helps kids get in touch with how intricate and intense their relationship with chemicals is.

28. Almost everybody thinks about suicide at one time or another. Do you? When? Ever think about it when you're high?

29. Have you ever tried suicide? What happened?

Note: If the student has suicidal thoughts, I look for any evidence that consideration of suicide is influenced by chemical use. If I find evidence, I usually get an immediate referral for assessment. For a detailed discussion of adolescent suicide, see *Suicide Attempts in Children and Youth* (McIntire and Angle, 1980).

30. How do your parents treat you?

31. Do you ever shift from one chemical to another? Why?

32. Do you avoid people who don't use?

33. Do you know what chemical dependency means? Ever talk about it?

34. Do you plan how much you're going to use? When to use?

35. Have you ever needed help when you're high or drunk? What happened?

36. When using have you ever done anything you were ashamed of? What happened?

37. Who is the most important person in your life, including yourself? What are you doing to take care of him or her?

38. On a scale of one to ten, how is your life going?

39. Can you think of any other consequences related to your chemical use besides those we have talked about?

Note: Questions 30 through 39 present an opportunity to review many of the consequences previously discussed. I find that these questions can be quite meaningful to the adolescent since we have usually broken down some defenses by this time in the interview.

40. Do you think your chemical use is harmful to you? Do you think you have a problem with chemicals?

Note: Recognition of even minor negative consequences related to use can be defined as a "problem." During the Insight Group, the adolescent's goal, then, is to become aware of how big the problem is and how much help is needed to deal with it.

When asking these questions, remember that the main considerations in conducting an Insight interview are: (1) Don't use it as an evaluation. (2) Try to make the experience a helpful one for the participant. (3) Make the interview an introduction to the Insight Group process by keeping in mind the goals of the Insight Group. (4) Help adolescents explore their relationship with chemicals and to see the consequences of their use. (5) Be ready to make decisions about levels of intervention if something other than an Insight Group is warranted.

If information is not readily forthcoming in the Insight interview, that does not mean that the student will not open up eventually.

Debbie is a case in point. She was very popular and involved in many extracurricular activities. She was referred to the Insight Group because of drinking at a school function. During the Insight interview she was defiant, discounted the interview process itself and minimized or made light of any data that indicated that she had used chemicals or had any trouble with chemical use. While in the Insight Group, she continued to manifest anger, especially when other students were talking about problems with their parents. She seemed to discount their experiences as insignificant and let them know that she could top all of them in regard to trouble with parents. The group helped her see that she did, in fact, have a lot of hostility toward her father and her father's drinking. That interaction with the group made her much easier to deal with and much more honest with me and the group.

Sometimes a person is very honest with me but very reticent in the group. In such cases, it is usually a simple matter to gently remind the student of some of the data he or she revealed to me in the Insight interview and to help him or her see how that data may tie into the issue being discussed in the group.

Confidentiality

Confidentiality is an ethical and professional issue as well as a legal one. Focusing exclusively on legal matters can be both misleading and counterproductive. Many schools begin a consideration of the confidentiality issue by bringing in a lawyer to explain the various laws applicable to confidentiality and to summarize past interpretations and future implications of those laws. It does not take much of a legal mind, however, to show teachers that they could be sued *for* revealing information that students tell them about their drug use and they could be sued *for not* revealing the same information when a student's life is in danger. Raising the possibility, however unlikely, of legalistic double binds only stimulates anxiety and does nothing to show staff members how to approach the issue of confidentiality in an ethical, professionally competent manner congruent with existing laws.

We do not mean to imply or promote a cavalier attitude concerning confidentiality. Sessions on confidentiality should be a regular part of any training program for all teachers, especially those working in an early-intervention program. School policies on confidentiality should be compatible in every respect with existing laws and regulations. For example, staff members should never talk publicly about confidential information or allude openly to a student's participation in an early-intervention program. And, of course, a counselor's written remarks about a student's behavior in a support group should never appear in that student's permanent record file.

We do want to stress that the great anxiety generated by the merest possibility of a lawsuit is unwarranted. Literally millions of students have attended schools with early-intervention programs without hostile legal action being taken by parents.

Confidentiality versus discretion

Some parents groups insist that school staff members who discover that a student is using drugs must immediately report this fact to the student's parents. However, if schools were forced to accede to this demand for immediate, automatic reporting (which is unlikely, since such a demand is probably incompatible with state and federal laws), the only option left to students would be to clam up with all school staff members. Thus, while proving their point about parental prerogatives, these parents could severely limit an early-intervention program's ability to identify and help young people with drug problems.

Allowing program staff members some discretion as to when they report a student's use of chemicals is advantageous for all involved. For instance, suppose a student in a support group reveals that he is using alcohol again; however, he is not totally out of control and does not appear to be in a life-threatening situation. Given time, the facilitator and the other students in the group could get him to see the consequences of his actions and persuade him to tell his parents that he is drinking again. Trust in the program would be maintained, and the student would have a chance to act responsibly on his own behalf.

Discretion vs. advocacy of "responsible use"

Some very effective counselors do not demand that a student who is just beginning individual counseling or has just joined an early-intervention group immediately agree to refrain from drug use. Does this stance constitute encouragement of "responsible use" of drugs? Hardly. There is a big difference between exercising some discretion in this matter and advocating responsible drug use.

Many staff members prefer to form an alliance with a young drug user before they demand an abstinence contract because they believe that without such rapport, the contract is meaningless. Their reasoning is simple: If the drug user has ignored school regulations, community norms and state and federal laws, he or she can hardly be expected to take another adult-imposed decree seriously. If, however, a counselor and a drug user have formed a healthy alliance, an abstinence contract can prove very meaningful, for it is then based on:

○ a shared perception that the young drug user is a person worthy of concern;

○ an agreement that drugs have been harmful in specific ways; and

○ an understanding that the purpose of counseling is to help, not to hurt or to discipline.

Important but nonconfidential information

In some school districts, student confidentiality is so closely protected that information revealed to a staff member can only be relayed to parents when the staff member judges the situation to be life-threatening. If this is the situation in your district, it may not be as much of an impediment as you may think. Much of the information needed to initiate an intervention is readily available to the school staff and parents and does not come from self-disclosure by the student. For example, a drop in grades, regular absenteeism and other observable behavioral cues do not fall under the jurisdiction of the laws on confidentiality. Often, such information is sufficient grounds for a school staff member to request an investigation of the problem. Furthermore, a counselor who has gained a student's trust can often persuade the student to tell parents about his or her drug use.

Consequences of being too confidential

In some schools, the rules on confidentiality are so strict that teachers cannot be told that a student is being treated for chemical dependency. Yes, of course, all the friends know. Yes, all the teachers will probably hear about it through the grapevine. Yes, the information will be distorted and in no way helpful in planning for a return to school after treatment. Such "confidentiality" fosters gossip and rumors, which perpetuate the stigma surrounding treatment and do nothing to help a young person in recovery.

Sharing information on a need-to-know basis only

To preserve a student's privacy, only those school staff members who *need* to know about the student's drug problems or other personal problems should have access to such information. When a student returns to school following treatment for a drug problem, for example, all the details do not have to be made known to all staff members. However, some teachers must be told about the classwork that the student completed while in treatment. Also, the general processes of a treatment group must be described to certain teachers if the student is to receive academic credit for participating in the group. In many other instances, it is to the student's benefit to share information and to the student's detriment if information cannot be shared. Most often, students themselves come to realize this and, with the support of a concerned adult, willingly share appropriate information with school staff members, parents and friends.

Let us reiterate. It serves no good purpose to "clarify" the issue of confidentiality by means of a legalistic, overly complicated debate. Staff members should be rigorously trained to protect students' rights in an appropriate fashion and to know when and how to share information. Those regulations or interpretations of regulations that appear to block early-intervention strategy should be changed, at the state level if necessary, to ensure that students are not shortchanged by bureaucratic caprice.

(Appendix B was adapted from *Alliance for Change* by James Crowley.)

Bibliography

Alcoholics Anonymous. Analysis of the 1980 survey of the membership of AA. New York: General Service Office of Alcoholics Anonymous, 1981

Anhalt H, Klein M. Drug abuse in junior high school populations. *American Journal of Drug/Alcohol Abuse* 1976;3:589-603

Benson PL, Wood PK, Johnson AL, et al. 1983 Minnesota survey on drug use and drug-related attitudes. Minneapolis: Search Institute, October 25, 1983

Biek JE, Screening test for identifying adolescents adversely affected by a parental drinking problem. *Journal of Adolescent Health Care* 1981;2:107-13

Booz-Allen and Hamilton, Incorporated. An assessment of the needs of and resources for children of alcoholic parents. Final report prepared for National Institute on Alcohol Abuse and Alcoholism. Springfield, VA: National Technical Information Service, November 30, 1974; grant No. ADM-41-74-0017

Borton T. A study of children's attitudes and perceptions about drugs and alcohol. Middletown, CT: Weekly Reader Periodicals of Xerox Education Publications, 1983

Bosma WG, Jensen P. Studies of approximately 500 children with behavior problems in the Baltimore area, 1972-1973. Unpublished research cited in Bosma WG. Adolescents and alcohol. In: Gallagher JR, Heald FP, Garrell DC, eds. Medical Care of the Adolescent. New York: Appleton-Century-Crofts, 1976

Bry BH, McKeon P, Pandina RJ. Extent of drug use as a function of number of risk factors. *Journal of Abnormal Psychology* 1982;91(4):273-9

Cohen AY, Santo Y. Youth drug abuse and education: empirical and theoretical considerations. In Beschner G, Friedman A, eds. Youth drug abuse. Lexington, Massachusetts: Lexington Books, D.C. Heath and Company, 1977

Cohn AH. Physical Child Abuse. Chicago: National Committee for Prevention of Child Abuse, 1983

Community Intervention, Inc. Demonstrating program effectiveness. *Community Intervention*, Fall 1982

Cooper DM, Olson DH, Fournier D. Adolescent drug use related to family support, self-esteem and school behavior. *Center for Youth Development and Research Quarterly*, Spring 1977. St. Paul: Center for Youth Development and Research, University of Minnesota

Cretcher D. Steering Clear: Helping Your Child Through the High-Risk Drug Years. Minneapolis: Winston Press, Inc. 1982

Crowley JF. Alliance for Change. Minneapolis: Community Intervention, Inc., 1984

Donovan JE, Jessor R. Adolescent problem drinking: psychosocial correlates in a national sample study. *Journal of Studies on Alcohol* 1978;39(9):1506-24

Egan G. The Skilled Helper: Model, Skills, and Methods for Effective Helping. 2nd ed. Monterey, CA: Brooks/Cole Publishing, 1982

Eliot TS. The hollow men. In: Collected Poems 1909-1962. New York: Harcourt, Brace & World, 1963

Gagnon J. Female child victims of sex offenses. *Social Problems* 1965;13:176-92.

Garfinkel BD, Froese A, Hood J. Suicide attempts in children and adolescents. *American Journal of Psychiatry* 1982;139(10):1257-61

Globetti G. Teenage drinking. In: Estes NJ, Heinemann ME, eds. Alcoholism: Development, Consequences, and Intervention. St. Louis: CV Mosby, 1977;162-73

Halikas JA, Lyttle MD, Morse CL, et al. Proposed criteria for the diagnosis of alcohol abuse in adolescents. *Comprehensive Psychiatry* 1984;25(6):581-5

Jellinek EM. The Disease Concept of Alcoholism. New Brunswick, NJ: Hillhouse Press, 1960

Johnson VE. I'll Quit Tomorrow. New York: Harper & Row, 1973

Johnston LD, Bachman JG, O'Malley PM. Student drug use in America, 1975-1981. Rockville, MD: National Institute on Drug Abuse, 1982(a); DHHS publication No. (ADM)82-1221

Johnston LD, Bachman JG, O'Malley PM. Student drug use, attitudes, and beliefs—national trends, 1975-1982. Rockville, MD: National Institute on Drug Abuse, 1982(b); DHHS Publication No. (ADM)83-1260

Johnston LD, O'Malley PM, Bachman JG. Drugs and American high school students, 1975-1983. Rockville, MD: National Institute on Drug Abuse, 1984; DHHS publication No. (ADM)85-1374

Kinsey AF. Sexual Behavior in the Human Female. Philadelphia: WB Saunders, 1953

Kite WR. Presenting problems of adolescents in treatment: a survey of CompCare adolescent programs. Newport Beach, CA: CompCare Corporation, Inc., December 1980

Larsen NE. Wayzata Chemical Health Program evaluation report. Unpublished report prepared for Wayzata Public Schools, Wayzata, MN, June 1982

Lennard HL, Epstein LJ, Bernstein A, et al. Mystification and Drug Misuse: Hazards in Using Psychoactive Drugs. San Francisco: Jossey-Bass, Inc., Publishers, 1971

Lowman C. Prevalence of alcohol use among U.S. senior high school students. Facts for Planning Series, No. 1. *Alcohol Health and Research World*, Fall 1981. Rockville, MD: National Institute on Alcohol Abuse and Alcoholism

Lowman C. Alcohol use as an indicator of psychoactive drug use among the nation's senior high school students. Facts for Planning Series, No. 2. *Alcohol Health and Research World*, Winter 1981/1982. Rockville, MD: National Institute of Alcohol Abuse and Alcoholism.

Mayer JV, Filstead WJ. The adolescent alcohol involvement scale: an instrument for measuring adolescent use and misuse of alcohol. *Journal of Studies on Alcohol* 1979;40(3):291-300

McIntire MS, Angle CR, eds. Suicide Attempts in Children and Youth. Hagerstown, MD: Harper & Row, 1980

McKinney JC. Constructive Typology and Social Theory. New York: Appleton-Century-Crofts, 1966

Mitchell J. St. Mary's Adolescent Treatment Program. Third-year final report, Hennepin County Drug/Alcohol Research Project, Minnesota. Minneapolis: Center for Planning and Research, Multi Resource Centers, Inc., December 1977; NIDA grant No. 1 H81 DA 01662-03

Muldoon JA, Berdie M. Effective Employee Assistance: A Comprehensive Guide for the Employer. Minneapolis: CompCare Publications, 1980

Namakkal S, Mangen DJ. Ninth-12th grade chemical use survey, 1979. Unpublished final report prepared for State of Minnesota, Department of Public Welfare, Prevention Branch, Chemical Dependency Program Division

National Institute on Alcohol Abuse and Alcoholism. Alcohol and youth. Alcohol Topics in Brief, November 1980; NIAAA publication code RP0067

National Institute on Alcohol Abuse and Alcoholism. Services for children of alcoholics. Research Monograph-4. Rockville, MD: National Institute on Alcohol Abuse and Alcoholism, 1981; DHHS publication No. (ADM)81-1007

O'Gorman PA, Lacks H. Aspects of youthful drinking. New York: National Council on Alcoholism, Inc., 1979

Omegon, Inc. Omegon self-assessment questionnaire: end of year report. Unpublished report. Minneapolis: Omegon Residential Treatment Center, March 1983

Pandina RJ, White HR, Yorke J. Estimations of substance use involvement: theoretical considerations and empirical findings. *International Journal of the Addictions* 1981;16(1):1-24

Pfeiffer JW, Jones JE. The 1973 Annual Handbook for Group Facilitators. Iowa City, Iowa: University Associates, 1973

Powell JJ. Why Am I Afraid to Tell You Who I Am? Chicago: Argus Communications, 1969

Rachal JV, Guess LL, Hubbard RL, et al. Alcohol misuse by adolescents. Facts for Planning Series, No. 4. *Alcohol Health and Research World,* Spring 1982. Rockville, MD: National Institute on Alcoholism and Alcohol Abuse

Rachal JV, Maisto SA, Guess, LL, et al. A national study of adolescent drinking behavior. Rockville, MD: National Institute on Alcohol Abuse and Alcoholism, 1980

Ray O. Drugs, Society, & Human Behavior. 3rd ed. St. Louis: CV Mosby, 1983

Rosenker D. The Chanhassen Adolescent Evaluation Unit: one year summary. Unpublished program data. Chanhassen, MN: Chanhassen Centers, 1982

Rusche S. How to form a Families In Action group in your community. Atlanta: Dekalb Families In Action, Inc., 1979

Sipe J, Hunter M. Minnesota Department of Corrections State Training School needs assessment, Unpublished paper, February 1980

Smart RG. Priorities in minimizing alcohol problems among young people. In: Blane HT, Chafetz ME, eds. Youth, Alcohol, and Social Policy. New York: Plenum Press, 1979; 229-61

Smart RG. The New Drinkers: Teenage Use and Abuse of Alcohol. Toronto: Alcoholism and Drug Addiction Research Foundation, 1980

Sullivan C. Child abuse in relation to chemical dependency and antisocial behavior. Unpublished research from Eden House Abuse Study. Minneapolis: Eden House, 1980

Vaillant GE, Milofsky ES. The etiology of alcoholism: a prospective viewpoint. *American Psychologist* 1982;37(5):494-503

Woodson AL. A method for identification of persons with problem-drinking parents. Paper presented at 27th annual meeting of the Alcohol and Drug Problems Association of North America, New Orleans, September 1976. Cited in Biek JE, 1981

Authors

Joseph A. Muldoon

Joseph A. Muldoon is a licensed psychologist with 14 years' experience in the treatment of and training on problems related to drug abuse. He is primary author of *Effective Employee Assistance*, published by CompCare Publications, Minneapolis, and editor of *Community Intervention*, the quarterly newspaper published by Community Intervention, Inc. He received his master's degree in psychology from the University of Minnesota and has worked as a psychologist for the Hennepin County Court system in Minneapolis and for the Jamestown Adolescent Chemical Dependency Treatment Center in Stillwater, Minnesota. He has also served as supervisor of counselors for Face-to-Face Health and Counseling in St. Paul and as a community organizer for VISTA in the southern United States.

James F. Crowley

James F. Crowley, president of Community Intervention, Inc., is author of *Alliance for Change: A Plan for Community Action on Adolescent Drug Abuse*. He is also executive producer of two 16 mm films: "A Better Place. . .A Better Time: Early Intervention Into Teenage Alcohol and Drug Problems" and "Open Secrets," a film about the reciprocal effects of communication problems and drug problems in a typical family.

Mr. Crowley earned a master's degree from St. Thomas College in St. Paul, Minnesota, and has ten years of teaching and administrative experience in both public and private schools. His career in drug intervention and prevention programming began in 1974, when he became executive director of the Johnson Institute in Minneapolis. He founded Community Intervention, Inc., in 1979.

Mr. Crowley has given hundreds of professional presentations to local community groups and to national organizations on the subject of community mobilization and early-intervention programs. He has also written articles on these subjects for numerous newspapers, magazines and professional journals.